Community-based Medical Education

a teacher's handbook

Edited by

LEN KELLY MD MClinSci FCFP FRRM
Professor, Northern Ontario School of Medicine
and Rural Physician

Foreword by
ROGER STRASSER AM FRACGP FACRRM FRCGP
Dean, Northern Ontario School of Medicine

Radcliffe Publishing
London • New York

Radcliffe Publishing Ltd
33–41 Dallington Street
London
EC1V 0BB
United Kingdom

www.radcliffepublishing.com

British Library Cataloguing in Publication Data

A catalogue record for this book is available from the British Library.

ISBN-13: 978 184619 505 1

Typeset by Phoenix Photosetting, Chatham, Kent, UK
Cover designed by Tracey Thomas
Printed and bound by Cadmus Communications, USA

Contents

Dedication

To Sharen
Always

Foreword

Community-based medical education (CBME) involves medical learners (students and residents/registrars) learning clinical medicine in community settings. The learners experience different social and clinical environments for themselves, rather than just learning about them in the classroom. Clinical learning sites may include mental health services, long-term care facilities and family practice clinics, as well as hospitals and health services in remote, rural and urban communities. CBME developed in the context of recognition that a relatively small proportion of the population are cared for in large acute teaching hospitals and that trends in healthcare are towards greater community-based care with tertiary-care hospitals focusing more on short-stay high-technology interventions for rare or serious, and often complex multi-system conditions.

For undergraduate medical education, the development of CBME in the 1980s and 1990s provided the basis for suggestions that students would benefit from prolonged community-based learning, specifically in family practice during which time the students learn their core clinical medicine known in North America as "clerkships." In the urban setting, this approach was developed at Cambridge in England and in rural family practice this approach was part of some "rural tracks" established by several US medical schools beginning in the 1970s. It was the Parallel Rural Community Curriculum (PRCC) of Flinders University in Australia which provided comprehensive research evidence of the value of rural family practice based CBME.

The Northern Ontario School of Medicine (NOSM), Canada's first medical school for the 21st century, was established in response to a chronic shortage of doctors and other health professionals in Northern Ontario, a geographically vast, sparsely populated part of the world. NOSM has taken CBME a step further with its own distinctive model of medical education and health research known as Distributed Community Engaged Learning (DCEL). DCEL weaves together: case-based learning; community-engaged education; learning in context; longitudinal integrated curricula; distributed learning; rural-based education; and integrated clinical learning. The NOSM curriculum is grounded in Northern Ontario and relies heavily on electronic communications to support DCEL. In the classroom and in clinical settings, students explore cases from the perspective of health professionals in Northern Ontario. In addition, DCEL involves community engagement through which communities actively partici-pate in hosting students and contribute to their learning.

Community-based Medical Education: a teacher's handbook has been developed by community-based educators for community-based educators. Len Kelly and his co-authors draw on research evidence and their collective experience to provide the reader with a wealth of practical knowledge about CBME. The authors build a bridge between educational principles and teaching in com-munity clinical settings. I expect that this book will be an invaluable resource to community practitioners with a teaching role whether they are new to teach-ing or have had learners in their practice for many years. In addition, this book will be useful to university-based educators who are seeking to assist clinical practitioners to be successful teachers.

For me, after over 30 years in medical education, it has been very refreshing to read this book and realize that I still have more to learn. It is written from the perspective of everyday clinical practice and provides helpful information on how to enhance the experience for the learners, the clinical teachers and the patients/community we have the privilege to serve.

I expect that *Community-based Medical Education: a teacher's handbook* will become a standard text in practice libraries and in medical schools around the world.

Roger Strasser AM, FRACGP, FACRRM, FRCGP
Dean and Professor
Northern Ontario School of Medicine, Canada
Former Head
Monash University School of Rural Health, Australia
September 2011

Introduction

Medical education is increasingly being distributed into community-based settings. As urban-based teaching centers continue their traditional role, there is a recognition that this specialized environment may not deliver role models for generalist models of care, particularly in rural areas. Additionally, university-based teaching facilities are becoming saturated and community-based options are being developed. These clinical teachers often may feel isolated and without teaching resources. We trust this manual will help address this.

Community-based medical education refers to comprehensive medical training which takes place in small communities under the clinical supervision of generalists. The term, therefore, encompasses rural training programs and those that occur in some intermediate-sized communities. We have included a chapter on inner city rotations since there are similar cultural and socio-economic challenges in the marginalized ranks of poor inner city community members. They share difficulty in accessing appropriate medical services in ways that differ from remote communities but pose similar challenges of care planning for their community physician.

Medical education has long been an anomaly. "See one, do one, teach one," an eternal standard describing the hands-on style of medical training which has been the norm. This apprenticeship model relies on direct access to the preceptor and speaks to the need for smaller learner groups, often hard to find in large teaching centers. The second assumption of this style of medical education is that one learns to teach by learning medicine, although teaching skills are secondary in the medical curriculum, if they are present at all.

This text is designed to give community-based medical educators a grasp of both some academic principles and the practical management of learners. The authors are all actively involved in teaching medical students and postgraduate residents in rural and urban environments. The chapters are stand-alone discussions of relevant topics supported with up-to-date scholarly references.

Categories of learners have been broadly divided into undergraduate and postgraduate. The latter designation refers to a variety of trainees in different constituencies: house officers, registrars and, more commonly, residents. Readers will have to be patient as we use variations of these terms throughout the text. Different jurisdictions construct their medical education along a wide range of designations. For example, international medical graduates in some settings will be employed in rural areas yet still under supervision and in training, while elsewhere they are residents in established postgraduate programs.

While primarily intended for clinical teachers of medicine, the principles and examples will be applicable to other healthcare professionals and non-medical teachers. Teaching skills can and often do develop in clinical teachers without much instruction by just finding a way, following the examples of their own teaching role models and using trial and error. A reference text such as this one may be useful when one encounters scenarios when tried and true methods do not work. Difficulty encountered in clinical teaching can put one off it altogether, since medical practice is one's main focus and teaching is optional. We recognize the stress teaching can add to a busy clinical load and hope that this book will support those who take on both duties. We have tried to "keep it simple." You will continue to encounter teaching scenarios for which even this text will not prepare you but hopefully it will help to orient clinical teachers along their career.

Len Kelly
September 2011

About the Editor

Len Kelly MD MClinSci FCFP FRRM, is a rural physician in Northern Ontario, Canada. He has spent his career involved in medical education and is a Professor in the Division of Clinical Sciences at the Northern Ontario School of Medicine in Sioux Lookout. He completed his undergraduate medical degree and Master of Clinical Sciences at the University of Western Ontario and family medicine residency at the University of Toronto. His on-going work includes a broad scope of rural medical practice and community-based education and research. He is a staff physician at the Sioux Lookout Meno Ya Win Health Centre.

Contributors

Ken Babey MD CCFP FRRM
Assistant Professor, University of Western Ontario and Rural Physician

David TS Barber MD CCFP
Assistant Professor, Department of Family Medicine, Queen's University and Regional Network Director, CPCSSN

Michael Betts MBBs Dip Obst RCOG FACRRM
Clinical Lecturer (Paediatrics) Flinders University Rural Clinical School and Rural General Practitioner

Michael Dillon MD CCFP FCFP
Assistant Professor, Family Medicine, University of Manitoba and Medical Director, Klinic Community Health Clinic

John Dove MDCM CCFP FCFP
Former Lecturer, Departments of Family Medicine, Queen's University, and McMaster University (retired) and Rural Physician

Blye Frank PhD
Dean, Faculty of Education, University of British Columbia

James Goertzen MD MClinSci CCFP FCFP
Associate Professor, Northern Ontario School of Medicine and Family Physician

Karen Hall Barber MD CCFP
Assistant Professor, Queen's University and Physician Lead, Queen's Family Health Team

Sasha Ho Ferris Nyriabu MD
Resident in Family Medicine, University of Manitoba and President of Canadian Association Interns and Residents

Keith MacLellan MDCM FRRM
Assistant Professor, Family Medicine, McGill University and Rural Physician

Anna MacLeod MA, PhD
Assistant Professor, Dalhousie University, NS, Canada

Aaron Orkin MD MSc CCFP
Lecturer, Northern Ontario School of Medicine and Family Physician

David Rosenthal MB BS Dip.RANZCOG FAMA FACRRM
Senior Lecturer and Assessment Coordinator, Flinders University Rural Clinical School, Rural Physician and Chief Consultant Safety & Quality Country Health SA

Leslie Rourke MD MClinSci CCFP FCFP
Associate Professor of Family Medicine, Memorial University of Newfoundland and Family Physician

James Rourke MD MClinSci CCFP (EM) FCFP LL
Professor of Family Medicine, Dean of Medicine Memorial University of Newfoundland

Yogi Sehgal MD CCFP FCFP FRRM
Assistant Professor, Northern Ontario School of Medicine and Rural Physician

Jeff Sloan MD CCFP FCFP
Assistant Professor, Family Medicine, Queen's University and Rural Physician

Karen Trollope-Kumar MD PhD
Assistant Professor, McMaster University and Co-director, Professional Competencies, Michael De Groote School of Medicine

David VanderBurgh MD CCFP
Resident in 3rd Year Family Medicine/Emergency and Locum Physician

Lucie Walters PhD MBBS DCH Dip RACOG FRACGP FACRRM
Associate Professor, Flinders University Rural Clinical School and Academic Director ACCRM

Susan Wearne BM MMedSci FRACGP FACRRM MRCGP DRCOG DFFP DCH GCTEd
Senior Lecturer in Clinical Educator Development, Flinders University Rural Clinical School, General Practitioner Alice Springs and Royal Flying Doctor Service Rural Women's Service, Ayers Rock Medical Centre, Northern Territory

Sandy Wells MSc
Senior Research Associate, Dalhousie University, NS

Ruth Wilson MD CCFP FCFP
Professor, Family Medicine, Queen's University and Family Physician

Community-based Medical Education

Len Kelly

Whether by default or design, medical education is arriving at distributed sites. Internationally, it has been recognized that rural and underserviced areas benefit little from a trickle-down effect of having medical education concentrated in urban areas. Students who spend time in community-based practices learn medicine which is tailored to care in that community without varying from quality, "standard of care" medical education. In fact, regional and national undergraduate exams from Canada and Australia show superior results in students with significant exposure to rural, community-based teaching sites, particularly in scores of clinical reasoning.

The involvement of medical learners in community settings occurs along a continuum. Tertiary care teaching hospitals send learners 'out' at various stages of training for short periods of time. The other end of the spectrum has learners in remote settings doing their complete medical training in their own region – now underway in the Northern Territories of Australia. Recently some medical schools in Canada and Australia send all of their students to rural areas to do their year-long clinical clerkships.

Students from community-based programs encounter a broad scope of patient concerns and also see the hardship that investigations and travel place on rural patients who prefer their care closest to home. Urban and rural community practices often introduce medical students to common primary care social issues which affect the patient's quality of life and the clinician's ability to offer care: poverty, addictions and family dysfunction. Rural placements offer incidental contact with patients outside of the office, rare in an urban setting. This highlights the challenge of physicians maintaining appropriate patient confidentiality and professional boundaries. In these communities, you are always a physician and, in a sense, always "on call." At the same time, the strengths and supports of the community as an extended family come to the surface. Learners experience the busy but interesting broad scope of medical practice available in rural community settings, as rural physicians often take on a variety of special skills that would otherwise be unavailable in the region. Inner city community practices are another "distributed site" where students often see patients with complex social and medical problems who navigate the medical system poorly and would otherwise "fall through the cracks." These patients, living on the geographic or social fringe, offer creative challenges for the community-based clinical teacher and their learner.

Primary care practices offer undifferentiated problems. These problems may attract a medical diagnosis or not. Functional, somaticized or behavioral complaints intermingle with initial presentations of serious disease. Undifferentiated disease is not commonly encountered in larger teaching centers, where patients may have been through an extensive triage and referral system. A wheezing adult may already have been identified as having reactive airways disease, congestive heart failure or chronic obstructive lung disease. The learner may know that, simply by knowing which specialized clinic the patient attends! The lack of this concentrating effect offers community-based practices the opportunity to teach learners skills in the identification and management of largely undifferentiated illness. The mixture of acute and chronic disease is the raw material of community practices. Learning the "red flags" of serious disease and the more sedate management of chronic illness are common required skills. Intertwined through all of these operations is the relationship with the patient and their community and culture, which both the clinical teacher and the learner must navigate.

If communication is the hallmark of the patient–doctor relationship, listening is its currency. Community-based clinical teachers' role model listening to all aspect of the patient's story, the one they already know from a long relationship with the patient and the developing illness script. They expose the learner to balancing between the medical detective and supportive nurturing roles common to physicians.

EDUCATIONAL CONTEXT
The Golden Rule

Community clinical teachers know it, but may not consciously acknowledge the golden rule: "patient care comes first." This is what distinguishes a clinical teacher from non-medical teachers. We are involved in an educational process with its attendant expectations of curriculum, evaluation and graduation. But our primary role is the appropriate relationship and medical management of our patients. This always takes priority over teaching. The learner's needs come second or even third. The educational context includes multiple relationships and responsibilities.

Relationships

Typically, a community-based clinical teacher is embedded into longstanding patient relationships that facilitate medical practice. The relationship with the patient is the cornerstone of their practice; the physician may have known the patient for years or even decades. They may resist the presence of a learner for fear they will compromise that important relationship, rather than enhancing it as the learner becomes involved.

The clinic setting is a key component of any practice. A lot of energy, thought and worry goes into it: hiring the right people, setting a common course, establishing collegial relations and creating a positive working environment. It is this setting which allows for the often arduous work of dealing with ill or troubled patients. A clinic setting does not arise *de novo* – it is actively nurtured. Into this mix of relationships and other duties comes the learner. They bring their anxieties, personalities, life experiences within and beyond medicine, as well as their learning tasks. How will they fit in? The learner begins a relationship with the teacher but also enters into all of the other intersecting connections as well. Learners with perceptive social skills pick that up intuitively; others may need more direct orienting.

Responsibilities

We have mentioned the learner's needs come second to the patient's, perhaps even third. The clinical teacher needs to be comfortable with the balance of clinical care, patient safety and educational oversight. That does not mean they sit back in a comfy chair while the work does itself. They need to be working within a real but ill-defined comfort zone. When a gravely ill patient challenges the physician to their limit, they may have little time or patience for the learner at that moment. A clinical teacher who has unusually stressful responsibilities on them on a given day (personal or professional) will have less energy or focus for the learner. These factors are a part of the day-to-day equation and the clinical teacher's comfort level will take precedence over their teaching role. These cards are on the table and all are in play, but not always consciously recognized. While a balance must be sought, there is a hierarchy of needs and the learners' will typically come after the patient's safety and the preceptor's comfort level. This does not lessen the importance of the educational agenda; rather it identifies its normal place in a clinical teacher's day. Conversely, it also highlights the need to put aside some purely educational time protected from heavy clinical responsibilities.

Social Accountability

No other medical training programs set the bar quite as high as rural training ones. They share the common educational requirement of graduating successful candidates. But rural programs are also judged by the subsequent work location of their graduates, a process they do not control. This is a very uncommon "educational" standard. Rural programs navigate the curriculum and competency challenges faced by all medical training initiatives. Not satisfied with this, we additionally define success as the development of rural physicians. This is a key outcome by which we measure training outcomes. Achieving this requires community engagement and developing distributed educational sites to expose learners to this interesting scope of practice.

Rural programs accept this added responsibility of contributing to needed physician manpower because their distant communities are so chronically underserviced. The rural physician manpower shortage is their regional context and by default and design becomes somewhat of a program imperative. This is truly applied social accountability. It is a realistic new standard by which to judge a medical education program. Monitoring vocational outcomes of graduates gives a transparent view of the feet-on-the-ground results underserviced areas require. It also gives programs meaningful community-relevant feedback from which educational and program adjustments can be made. Contributing appropriately to the rural workforce is both the community and evidence-based gold standard by which rural training programs are judged. Rural preceptors welcome this scrutiny. Successful recruiting of well-trained graduates is a high priority for their communities and their own careers.

MEDICAL EDUCATION AS A SOCIALIZATION PROCESS

I smile when I hear casualty patients appear relieved when I tell them they have a fracture: "Whew, at least it's not broken," they say. I can recall before medical training, that indeed something that was fractured was not as bad as a break, although now they are the same thing. It points out to me the different language and thinking process we now use as physicians.

The language we use is, of course, an extension of our conceptual framework and paradigms. What other subtle (or not so) changes have we undergone? We likely see ourselves more as a worker bee than as part of the establishment. Our patients may not share that perspective and may have us on a pedestal.

Learning medicine is a real, but poorly documented socialization process. As clinical teachers, we are embedded in that reality while our learners are just entering the process. What role does that play in the gap between us? We share that we are both still learning, but the teacher has advanced far along the disease recognition process, which set us apart and renders us the expert.

In many ways, the learner wants to be like us. They usually want to "please" us. They expend energy learning the unspoken rules for a given rotation. And the rules change with every rotation and each teacher. This can be a stressful process for the learner. It certainly takes a lot of their energy. They want to make a good impression, fit in, be liked and receive a reasonable evaluation. We need to acknowledge that process, even if we do not consciously do anything about it. Learners juggle these diverse tasks and it changes them. Medical educational research consistently identifies that student empathy measurably decreases during their clinical clerkship year. We need to keep this untoward effect in mind as educators. Do we portray empathy in our patient care, in our dealings with learners? Whether we acknowledge it or not, we are role models. Our behavior counts. Good will counts. Treat every learner as if they are potential recruits to your practice and your future colleagues.

Create a positive learning environment, but deal with learning issues as they arise. Students want to learn how we think. Recognizing congestive heart failure, because you have seen it numerous times, or because you know the patient's history may be easy for us, but is a giant leap for a learner. They are looking at different cues. They are trying to look intelligent to their preceptors and dealing with a sick patient, while simultaneously trying to integrate what they have learned in the classroom to arrive at a diagnosis. It is quite a handful but somehow we all seem to get through it. Explaining how we think and arrive at our working diagnoses is very useful to the learner. Sharing that process with them de-mystifies some of medicine for them, but also demonstrates our cognitive processes and the mental equations we perform without even knowing it. The socialization and learning process is behavioral, attitudinal and cognitive. Since the learner is the nearby sponge, we should try to be at our best.

MEDICAL EDUCATION THEORY

Education and medicine are two very different fields. Medical education in community-based clinical supervision is not a melding of the two but remains largely undescribed theoretically. Very little evidence supports one established educational method over another. Systematic reviews and meta-analyses typically show limited superiority of one over another method of medical education. Problem-based learning underwent systematic review in 1993 and 2002 and, despite its widespread use, had little benefit above traditional didactic methods of instruction and learning. Most proponents of one method's superiority are case reports or opinion pieces. Leung and Johnston pointed out in a 2006 review that evidence-based standards may never be brought to bear on our approach to education due to four limitations: medical schools already undergo rigorous accreditation regularly and may not welcome further scrutiny; it is difficult to describe and agree on the outcome of interest: exam passing, successful clinical careers; it would be expensive to study and all schools are context-rich small samples which might not combine meaningfully.

One recent educational advancement is competency-based evaluation. This affects community-based preceptors as it requires assessment by observation of the learner's application of their knowledge and skills. This is a good initiative and it requires us to observe the learner with a patient and document it. It is a task we often like to avoid, but it does allow us to see for ourselves how the learner handles themselves with patients and give them useful feedback.

So, during our careers, approaches will come and go. Justification may be found in some quarter for a given method, as long as learners continue to pass their qualifying exams. Be reassured that no theory is a panacea. Remain confident in your developing teaching skills and familiarize yourself with the shifting program requirements as required. Community-based teachers will be at arms' length for much of this process due in part to the primacy of clinical care of patients and a healthy distance from the university. Like most things in our busy practice, we will use what works in our setting and move forward. Community-based preceptors must be active participants in the development of relevant curriculum and exam questions whenever they can. We also need to comply with evaluation and monitoring guidelines supplied by the programs. Aside from that, we are on our own. The good thing about that is that we can be creative in our clinical teaching. The downside is that areas in which we are weak (typically feedback and evaluation) may remain weak unless we supplement them. We are unlikely to read medical education journals as we can barely keep up with our medical ones. That leaves faculty development sessions as our likely source of educational development. These programs must welcome community-based clinicians into their midst and need to be given locally or be conveniently added onto conferences already frequented by preceptors. Availability on stored digital webcasts is another developing continuing education technology.

Generally we will learn from our peers, students, educational success stories and failures. An apprenticeship model is still the hallmark of community-based medical education and remains its strength. The clinical teacher and learner are on the same side of the equation. The other side includes excellence in patient care and on-going learning (*see* Figure 1.1).

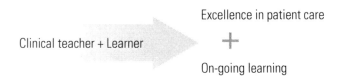

Clinical teacher + Learner

Excellence in patient care

$+$

On-going learning

Figure 1.1 A Teaching, Learning and Patient Care Team

LEARNING AND TEACHING

We spend our career doing both. One affects the other in unknown ways: learning and teaching. By supervising learners, we acknowledge they keep us up-to-date with their questions and expectations. As we become more experienced in teaching, we master more of it, often by trial and error. Our teaching skills will grow over time, as we become less nervous when giving presentations or become less rattled when facilitating a small group session. The amount of medical knowledge we accumulate grows but the rate likely declines as we focus on upgrading certain skills while relying on others that have been consolidated. So, our learning and teaching travel with us in our career. For career-long community-based medical educators, they are both a part of what medicine is for us. Teaching and learning jointly contribute to our quality of professional life, quality of patient care and our enjoyment of each.

Are there phases where one aspect moves at a different pace to the other? What does a career of learning and teaching look like over time? I suggest some predictable phases of each below (*see* Figure 1.2).

Phase 1

Generally called "clinical clerkship," this time is often clustered in a year-long series of clinical rotations with discrete learning objectives and evaluations. The learning slope is uphill and quite challenging. These novice clinicians are exposed to working alongside expert clinicians. These experts are experienced at clinical pattern recognition, disease symptoms clustering and spot diagnoses. There is a considerable communication and knowledge assimilation gap to be bridged by measured and comprehensive communication between the learner and their clinical teacher. Clinical clerks want to learn and they also want to fit in. One of the dangers of this is that they will go with the flow of patient diagnosis and treatment without fully understanding, or worse, with incorrect assumptions about diagnosis and treatment. Not fitting in and not being assumed to be stupid are often a clerk's greatest fear. This is a time for taking huge steps in learning how to think as a clinician. This is also the beginning of one's teaching career. Clerks do some short topic and case presentations from time to time and will see how difficult it is to "keep it short." It is a useful time for them to be taught some rudimentary presentation skills.

Phase 2

These are residency years. Here we may enjoy the steepest learning curve and most stimulating learning environments in our career. It may even be the steepest slope on the learning curve and even a learning high-point of a career. Graded clinical responsibilities, coupled with clinical supervision and backup, are ideal impetus to learning. Encouraged to develop diagnostic and treatment plans, interns and residents are able to put their earlier acquired knowledge to use. This is where it counts, as their orders will be implemented and will affect patient care. Given appropriate supervision and "checking" of treatment (including actually changing it), the educational rubber meets the road in a safe manner.

Teaching capacity is quite good here. The new resident is not far removed from the undergraduate experience. They know how confusing clinical scenarios can be, as well as how to navigate the medical politics of venturing onto the hospital wards. Protected time for teaching small groups of medical students is often the norm. What is often missing is a series of seminars on how to teach: how much to cover, how to approach it, how to facilitate small group discussions and be encouraging. It is an ideal time for educational resources to be invested in the resident, who may eventually be a life-long learner and teacher. If you are a staff member delegating these teaching responsibilities to a resident, part of your responsibility is to ensure the resident is provided with access to these skills, or advise them yourself.

Phase 3

This is the early independent physician. The buck has stopped – it has stopped here. The weight of being a clinician is undertaken. Aside from the medical responsibilities come emotional, professional, personal financial and even community roles and responsibilities. This is often our time of most up-to-date knowledge. Even as a generalist, we recall the paradigms used throughout the specialty rotations we have just completed. We know to whom and how to refer patients requiring specialty assessment, as well as how their primary care management should be handled.

Surprisingly, this is generally a time of limited teaching capacity at this juncture, despite being a potential fount of clinical information. Entering or beginning a practice is a consuming endeavor, and there may not be enough reserve energy to dedicate to a learner. A 6–24 month reprieve from teaching responsibilities is safe practice – but perhaps not required by all. It is a wonderful time to be exposed to the teaching practices of your more long-standing colleagues, while you deal with the practical issues of learning the management of a clinical practice. You will know when you are ready to take on learners and may develop better teaching habits if you can bring an appropriate amount of energy to initiating the process.

Phase 4

A wizened or experienced clinician who has now dealt with many similar presenting problems will have dealt with uncertainty and often developed an approach to problems which work in their particular setting. They possess a strong ability to teach simplifying the patient information into "serious" and "not serious," "treatable" and "not treatable;" recognize the importance of the joining of patient and clinician in finding common ground; have long-standing communication experience; can add the art to the science of medicine; can talk of mistakes made and how they were approached; can attest to their limitations and how we will encounter such limitations throughout our career; may not always have the most up-to-date clinical approach but will have supporting strategies for finding out and getting there safely.

Longevity here is enhanced by an active learning strategy of continuing medical education and by working in a group setting of up-to-date peers. Personal health concerns diminish both teaching and learning capacities.

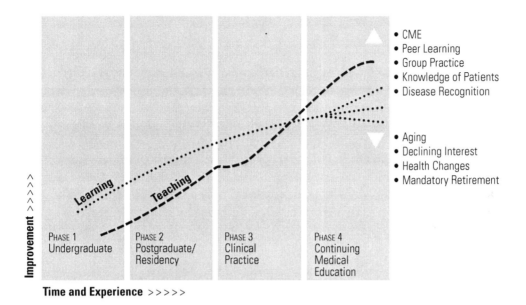

Figure: 1.2 A Career of Learning and Teaching

These phases may seem familiar to some and may follow a divergent course for many others. It is interesting to speculate when we have been, or will be, at our best clinically and educationally. We may be satisfied with our course or may want to make adjustments.

FURTHER READING

Haidet P. Jazz and the "art" of medicine: improvisation in the medical encounter. *Ann Fam Med.* 2007; 5(2): 164–9.

Walters L, Greenhill J, Ash J, et al. *Longitudinal Clinical Placements: time for a theoretical framework.* 2011, in press.

2

Contracting

Len Kelly

This is often overlooked and teaching programs rarely mention it but it is very important. When a learner arrives, the clinical teacher may show them around or an office manager may do so: the washroom, lunchroom and the coffee pot! A welcome is in order. This is a very stressful first meeting for the learner. They are starting a new rotation. Welcome and reassure them. Even if you are in the middle of seeing patients, take a bit of time. If there is not a lot of time in the morning, the rest of the contracting session can be done at the end of the day. Beyond the welcome, educational contracting involves making two things explicit: the expectations of the teacher and program and the learner's needs.

PATIENT SAFETY

Many clinical teachers think the student knows what is expected of them. They may not. This is our time to tell them. What are the time responsibilities and constraints? Are they expected to follow admitted inpatients on the weekends? Are the program requirements clear to each of them? This is the time to tell the learner how the flow of patients, pressure and information goes.

Also, it is an important time to go over the golden rule: patient care and safety come first. This means that if the learner feels out of their depth or uncomfortable with a given patient or procedure, they are to stop and get help. The learner is here to learn and I am here to work. Specifically, the learner must know how and when to get hold of the preceptor. Finding out later that "I didn't want to bother you" or "I didn't know if I should interrupt you" after something has gone wrong is very problematic.

PRECEPTOR EXPECTATIONS

There is a well-established concept in medical education called "graded responsibility." As a learner progresses through their training, they know more and can be delegated more responsibility. The preceptor always does oversight: for a beginner, every patient they see must also been seen by the teacher. Did they get the story right? Is there an obvious emotional or cultural overlay they have missed? The initial contracting session is a time to let the learner know where you see them fitting into this graded responsibility gradient. This varies from service to service and depends on the level and competence of the learner and the gravity of the clinical problem. Can they send a patient home or do you need to see them? Does the treatment need to be discussed before the patient leaves or can it wait until the end of the day? Clearly this will need to evolve over a short period of time as teacher and learner find their joint comfort level. But a discussion of patient and learner safety and expected supervisory practices should take place in advance.

A more senior learner will see patients on their own, with easy access to their supervisor, and will go over patient management later that day. This is graded responsibility. It needs to be adapted to each learner. A novice will begin by "puppy-dogging," merely following the teacher around. Once comfortable with doing a patient interview on their own, they may do so. In contrast, a senior learner is expected to already have those skills, but may not, and they may need to start at an earlier stage of more supervision rather than less.

These practical preceptor considerations can be elaborated during a contracting session to help the learner understand their clinical role.

LEARNERS' EXPECTATIONS

In fact, most learners will not express particular learning needs, but it is important to encourage them to identify any deficits they may have in their expertise or in their previous clinical exposure. I let them know that this is one of the few times in their career where they are encouraged to look at areas of deficiency and improve on them. We all like to deal to our strong suit and learners are no different. I tell them that things I learned poorly during my training have sometimes remained weak areas throughout my career!

I often ask about specific skills required for community-based medicine: appropriate history taking, physical examination skills, including gynecology and rectal examinations. More generally, if the learner has a sense of what branch of medicine interests them, we can try to plan an exposure to it for them, keeping in mind that things change and they will need to encounter a broad exposure during their educational process. Learners who never plan to deliver babies may find they love it. Any aversion to a given area of medicine is not an opportunity to avoid it during the rotation, and that needs to be made clear to learners. If the learner has a specific interest, then we try to accommodate that with a balance of curriculum and practice requirements.

This is also an obvious time to find out about any absences they plan for holidays, conferences or other approved activities. If they have program requirements for a research project at some point in time, discussing it early in a rotation gives time to develop the idea and even gather data during the time together. It is also a time to see if there are any other considerations requiring time away from the coming workload, like personal or family responsibilities or plans.

DOCUMENTATION

This can all be done very informally, but on-call expectations need to be made clear to each party. A simple note in the student's file documenting the session is also appropriate. If contentious issues arise in the initial session, document the session with what has been agreed upon. This is rare and speaks to the likelihood of a challenging experience ahead for both learner and preceptor. If team hierarchies exist (consultant, fellow, senior resident etc.), any expectations along the chain of responsibility must be made clear to the learner upon orientation. In community-based scenarios, these are less and it is typically the preceptor who is directly responsible for both patient care and learner supervision. Programs may have their own stated expectations, and how they are achieved may differ from town to town as well as between practices.

ORIENTATION: SET A WELCOMING TONE

A recent survey of New York internal medicine residents found many of them were already burned out upon starting their residency. A 2005 study of family medicine residents in Ontario showed that 8% of them would take a mental health leave of absence during their 2-year program.

So, we need to be aware that our learners bring their baggage. We need not onerously add to it on day one. Giving them an encouraging welcome, clarifying their role and responsibilities and facilitating two-way communication is a good start.

If they have arrived during the clinic day, only some of that will be accomplished on the spot, with the rest at the end of the day. After clinic, a tour of the town is generally in order. Other than the location of the grocery store and other amenities, we need to orient the student to the location of the hospital, old-age home and any other locales in which they will have clinical duties. Sometimes, a brief document describing the clinic practices and any specific clinical opportunities (e.g. fracture clinic, stress-testing) is helpful.

That is usually enough for day one. The next day, we generally meet at the hospital and carry out rounds. Beyond meeting the patients, this is a good time to make introductions to the nurses and other physicians and clerical staff. The learner needs to be and feel a part of the treatment team. If time permits, a brief incursion into how the medical charts work is in order. If electronic medical records are the standard, then an appointment with the appropriate medical records person can be set up.

If the learner is senior and will be carrying more clinical responsibilities, greater care needs to be taken in facilitating a comfort level within the hospital setting. Where there is more responsibility, there will be increased stress for the learner, and we need to play a role in lessening that. If the learner does not already know it, now is the time to say that the nurses will always call the preceptor first is there is a dire emergency, and that they are not expected to cover life-threatening emergencies on their own. This is a big fear for learners in community-based practices and needs to be explicitly clarified.

SUMMARY

Contracting is the beginning of the student–teacher professional relationship. It gives each party an opportunity to place their cards on the table. If there is a hidden curriculum, this is a good time to clarify it somehow. At the beginning of a relationship, a positive note is best and laying the groundwork for on-going communication and troubleshooting is important. The learner needs to clearly understand your expectations; these may need reinforcement in the days to come. It does not have to be done in one, often overwhelming session, but can be done through after-clinic chats over the first few days. Look at it as an investment in problem prevention and opening solid lines of communication. It is time well spent.

FURTHER READING

Earle L, Kelly L. Depression, anxiety and coping strategies in Ontario family medicine residents. *Can Fam Phys.* 2005; **51**: 243.

Hoff T, Pohl H, Bartfield J. Creating a learning environment to produce competent residents: the roles of culture and context. *Acad Med.* 2004; **79**(6): 532–9.

Kelly L. Integrating a family medicine resident into a rural practice. *Can Fam Phys.* 1997; **43**: 277–86.

Pratt D, Macgill M. Educational contracts: a basis for effective clinical teaching. *J Med Educ.* 1983; **58**: 462–7.

Raszka W, Maloney C, Hanson J. Getting off to a good start: discussing goals and expectations with medical students. *Pediatr.* 2010; **126**(2): 193–5.

Ripp J, Fallar R, Babyatsky M, *et al.* Prevalence of resident burnout at the start of training. *Teach Learn Med.* 2010; **22**(3): 172–5.

3

Monitoring

Len Kelly

We work shoulder to shoulder with the learner and assume we know how they interact with patients. But do we? There is no replacement for observing how that interaction actually transpires. How else will we know if the learner appears rude, impatient, establishes eye contact, listens appropriately to the patient's concern? Many medical education programs now require monthly documented observation sessions.

There are high-tech and low-tech means of monitoring. Each has its pros and cons. The key thing is not to let the method interfere with the goal: observation of the patient–learner interaction accurately and unobtrusively. As with all educational pursuits, patient care and safety come first. Some methods might work better with some patients while others may cause concern. Patient consent is always required. Tacit consent may begin with signs in the waiting room stating that this is a teaching practice and that students will be involved in their medical care. However, for observed sessions, explicit and specific consent will be needed.

OVERVIEW

Assessing medical knowledge is generally accomplished by multiple-choice and short-answer questions. However, history, physical examination, communication skills and professionalism need to be seen to be believed. Observation of learners can be direct (sitting in on the patient consultation) or indirect (audio- or videotaping). It can occur with actual or simulated patients, in the office, hospital or exam setting. It is important to cover a range of patient presentations and management scenarios during the course of the rotation.

Even though monitoring by observation is the key to assessing much of what we want our students to learn, it is often neglected. A 2004 survey of 97 Canadian and American pediatric programs found only 56% of the clinical clerkships rotations included direct observation. One year later, a similar survey of 109 North American internal medicine programs noted only 22% of their clinical clerks were directly observed.

The response of some medical education programs has been the development of regular direct observation requirements of their students, even when in community rotations. This is a healthy obligation and needs supplementation by accompanying faculty development. Assessment tools will often be provided to the community preceptor to allow a "scoring" of history, physical, communication skills and professionalism. Organized summative exams called Objective Structured Clinical Exams (OSCEs) or Simulated Office Orals (SOOs) are becoming commonplace. Aside from these somewhat formalized initiatives, community-based clinical teachers may need to know how direct and indirect observation can be accomplished in their own practice. We shall look at how observation monitoring can work well in community settings.

DIRECT OBSERVATION MONITORING

"Fly on the Wall"

This is the simplest, yet sometimes most challenging, type of monitoring. It can easily be introduced into any practice. If we consider the typical clinic setting: a junior learner goes in to see the patient on their own and then returns with their preceptor who verifies the history and relevant physical examination, while a senior learner will see the patient on their own, and if there is no obligation or need to simultaneously consult the preceptor, the patient is treated, discharged and a management "chart review" is done case by case at the end of the day.

In order to directly observe each of these learners with a patient, some planning is necessary. The caseload needs to be specifically light that afternoon. In the case of a senior learner, the patient is booked to see them. They go in and introduce themselves to the patient and ask if Dr. Smith, their clinical supervisor, might participate in the dialogue. If the patient declines, the resident proceeds as they usually would. This rarely occurs, but might if the patient does not want to see that particular preceptor or may be in a rush. Typically, the patient agrees and the resident goes and brings back the preceptor-observer. At this point, everyone is a bit nervous. Relax, this is normal and will quickly settle.

The preceptor enters the room with the senior learner who has gone to fetch them after getting the patient's permission. Alternately, if the patient has been booked to see the preceptor (as with a junior learner) the preceptor will ask permission since the care "contract" is with them. The preceptor thanks the patient for allowing them in as an observer and sits in a pre-arranged corner. It is important that the preceptor does not engage in eye contact with the learner or the patient after the initial greeting. What usually happens is that as the learner asks a question, the patient will turn and direct their answer to the preceptor, with whom they are more familiar. This deferential behavior toward the preceptor will continue, if it is sustained by reciprocal eye contact from the preceptor. You are a "fly on the wall" and this is a new role for you. If the preceptor literally focuses on looking at their blank note page or turns expectantly toward the learner, the patient will eventually begin to focus on the learner. In a very short time, the observer is forgotten. Until you have done this, you will have no idea of how well it works. The obstacles are actually preceptor based. They feel it might be rude – it certainly is unusual – to avoid eye contact with the patient and to not respond to their question. This is more the case when it is a patient you may know well. The second preceptor-based obstacle is impatience. It is challenging for an experienced interviewer and clinician to sit silently while listening to a slowly paced interview by a developing clinician. The urge to "take over" the interview must be resisted unless it compromises patient comfort or care parameters.

While the interview progresses, the preceptor can take verbatim notes of key questions by the learner or comments by the patient. The preceptor and learner may have to leave the room if the patient needs to undress. More invasive physical exam components will need to be negotiated with the patient and the learner as the need arises, relying on the preceptor's judgment and patient preference. The learner then concludes the exam and they can then discuss the medical assessment and treatment plan in front of the patient or adjourn to the office and discuss it with the preceptor.

Once the patient problem has been concluded, and the medical treatment and follow-up has been arranged, the patient is thanked for allowing an observed session and departs. The preceptor and learner can then go over the interaction, allowing for timely feedback. This requires a gap in patient booking to allow for this, before the next patient arrives.

Direct observation is a bit nerve-wracking for the learner. When the patient has left, I ask the student how that was. "How did that feel?" Often, they need to take a deep breath and state that they were nervous. Remember, we are combining the challenge of patient care with the stress of observation! This high emotional content will decrease as more direct observations occur. Finding out how that felt for the learner, aside from a typical case of nerves, will also touch on any occurrences of transference: that patient made me feel sad or angry. Once that part of discussion has concluded, I ask how the session went. Most of us are our most severe critics. If the interview in fact went poorly, the preceptor can merely agree with the learner's appraisal and comment that they have good self-monitoring skills. The preceptor can now refer to their notes and read back insightful or awkward phrases to the student. They will often not even recall using them, so it is useful to have actual quotes. We often use phrases that have a certain meaning for ourselves, but are open to misinterpretation by others, particularly non-physicians or patients with different educational levels.

Once the debriefing is done, move on to the next patient. Keep some "field notes" about each interaction. They can be included in the student's file. I usually document the type of patient and their complaint and then how the learner did and what educational aspects we discussed.

One-way Mirror Observation

This may be a middle position between low- and high-tech. The advantage (and part of the problem) is that the preceptor may be doing other things at the same time as observing the learner–patient interaction. Their attention is not totally focused on observing the student, as it is in direct observation. The room needs a closure system to prevent the one-way mirror always being in use. This should be on the patient side, so they know it is not in use. The same should hold for any audiotaping equipment. The patient should be able to know that it is not in use.

Observed interviews with this system require the same attention to documenting behaviors and words for later discussion. If the interview needs to be altered by the preceptor, a telephone call to the room can be used. Using an overhead intercom system will feel quite foreign to the patient and the learner. This system is direct observation, and feedback would proceed as in the scenario where the preceptor is in the exam room with the patient and learner.

Typical Direct Observation Issues

Patterns can be seen in the type of deficits learners have at different training levels. Junior students are steeped in history-taking, which is where they feel safest. When you ask them what they think might be wrong with the patient, they give more historical information. It is very predictable. They keep returning to the patient's history, as if you might be satisfied with more of that. Commenting on diagnosis is challenging for them, even if asked in the most non-threatening manner. During the observed session, you will see the junior learner take an inordinate amount of time and detail in history-taking. That is to be expected, as that is where they are most comfortable at this point in their development.

More experienced learners may be more diagnosis focused and they are more likely to neglect open-ended questions at the beginning of the interview. Be alert as to the openness of the initial questions asked by the learner. You will be surprised how quickly the learner falls into a more comfortable pattern of closed-ended questions. By doing this, they have nudged the interview into a set of predictable questioning which flows between one another. If they have actually missed the reason for the consultation, these questions lead to a dead end. It is then hard for the novice interviewer to notice that they, essentially, need to start all over again with more open-ended questions.

The beginning of the learner–patient interview should include multiple open-ended questions allowing the patient to fully describe their concerns, but it often does not. Most learners are uncomfortable with uncertainty and feel they need to get to a "diagnosis" to be efficient, appear clever and please their preceptor. Jotting notes as to what questions were asked at the beginning of the interview is usually very fruitful, as you can document how few open-ended questions were actually asked. Typically, even an experienced learner will ask only one or two open-ended questions at the beginning of an interview. They become uncomfortable with uncertainty, particularly as they are being observed, and retreat to closed-ended questioning. It can be a very valuable feedback session for the learner. You can repeat back to them how the interview began. Commonly, you will be pointing out to them additional open-ended questions that may have been helpful to really understand why the patient was there. This senior learner is beginning to experience what all junior doctors confront; uncertainty. What they need to learn is to hang in with open-ended questions until the pathway to the patient complaint is clearly established by the patient. I have seen these two patterns of interview scenarios consistently over the years: student comfort with history-taking and resident discomfort with uncertainty and open-ended questioning.

Ending the interview requires "coming out of the role" for the preceptor. The learner is encouraged to end the interview when they have reached the allotted time limit or have concluded their assessment and treatment of the presenting problem. The learner then turns to the "wallflower" observer and asks if they have any questions. If the preceptor and the learner do not have a handle on things clinically, the preceptor will encourage other lines of enquiry by the learner or just ask themselves. This is when patient care trumps educational priorities and so that the consultation can be concluded in a timely and satisfactory fashion. Once the session has concluded debriefing can occur. Sometimes the patient is only in for a brief assessment of pharyngitis and the interaction is simple and brief. That is fine, move on. Three to four direct-observed patient encounters on a given afternoon is plenty, as this can be tiring for both parties.

We will go into the elements of feedback in Chapter 4. For completeness, this how a short and direct debriefing might go:

> "How did that go, how did you think that interview went?"
> "What do you think you did well?"
> "What could have gone better? How? Why?"
> "What could you have done differently?"
> "During the interview:
>   You used these words
>   You performed the exam in this manner
>   Your body language, tone of voice was…"
> "Is that what you were trying to portray?"

"What meaning might the patient ascribe to that?"
"Do you have any other comments?"
"Good, let's see the next patient."

INDIRECT OBSERVATION
Video-monitoring

This was very popular when it was first introduced several decades ago and is still commonly used. Community offices were given video equipment by university centers, often without any instruction of how it can be used to best educational advantage. In the right hands, it can be an excellent teaching and learning tool. Consent for filming needs to be received from the patient. The use of the taped record has to be clear to the patient. If the tape will become a permanent teaching tool, formal written patient consent should be obtained.

There is a slight pedagogic dilemma in how videotaping can be used to best advantage. Feedback should be given in a timely fashion, as soon after the interaction as possible. Learners, however, may have a powerful learning experience if they have the time to view and evaluate their own interviews, before receiving any feedback. They then see and hear for themselves the body language and the type of questions they used. This occurs without the intervention or layer of the preceptor's intercession and can be a powerful learning experience.

A compromise may be that the preceptor gives feedback of a videotape either by watching it "live" or after it is done and the learner views it on their own time and comes to conclusions about its strengths and weaknesses before they discuss it.

Sometimes the set-up allows for synchronous monitoring by the preceptor, allowing for them to not be in the room, but still give accurate feedback and evaluation directly after the session, even before the patient leaves. If that is not possible, then video-monitoring may not be suitable for the novice learner who cannot be delegated independent patient care duties.

Educational programs can often provide "patient-actors" with standard roles and presenting problems. If these are available to come to your community practice, take advantage of the offer. These standardized patients become very accomplished in their roles and sometime naturally respond to the engaging or off-putting interviewer. If local theatre groups are available, they make an obvious resource for such roles in small communities. Otherwise, practices may develop their own scenarios and role-play in a more simple fashion.

All of these can also lend themselves to video-monitoring observation. When the tape is viewed with a resident, the debriefing can proceed as outlined above. Rather than quoting particular parts of the interview, the resident or preceptor can access sections of interest to them. The tape can be rewound to the appropriate section. Obviously, this requires familiarity with use of the equipment. The challenge is to get to the heart of the learner–patient interaction and not become side-tracked by playing around with the equipment! If the tape is to be kept in a teaching file, its storage must respect patient confidentiality. This may not always be possible in a small community-based practice, where clinic staff and other physicians may be related to or know the patient socially.

Establishing trust and respect with patients who are members of a minority culture is a critical part of rendering appropriate medical care. Certain cultures may also take issue with videotaping or other non-direct forms of observation. This will need to be explored within each practice norms and even with each patient. As with all medical care, confidentiality must be ensured and patient care comes before educational duties.

SUMMARY

Monitoring is typically an underused but important aspect of medical education. Whichever system is adopted, it should be a good fit for the clinical practice and become routine for both the community-based preceptor and their learners.

FURTHER READING

Bellet PS. How I teach medical students as an attending physician. *Med Teach*. 1992; 14(2): 231–9.

Craig S. Direct observation of clinical practice in emergency medicine education. *Acad Emerg Med*. 2010; **18**: 1–8.

Dattner L, Lopreiato J. Introduction of a direct observation program into a pediatric resident continuity clinic: feasibility, acceptability and effect on resident feedback. *Teach Learn Med*. 2010; **22**(4): 280–6.

Hanson J, Bannister S, Clark A, *et al.* Oh, what you see: the role of observation in medical student education. *Pediatr*. 2010; **126**(5): 843–5.

Hauer K, Holmbes E, Kogan J. Twelve tips for implementing tools for direct observation of medical trainees' clinical skills during patient encounters. *Med Teach*. 2011; **33**(1): 27–33.

Hemmer P, Paap K, Mechaber AJ, *et al.* Evaluation, grading and use of the RIME vocabulary on internal medicine clerkships: results of a national survey and comparison to other clinical clerkships. *Teach Learn Med*. 2008; **20**(2): 118–26.

Kumar A, Gera R, Shah G, *et al.* Student evaluation practices in pediatric clerkships: a survey of the medical schools in the United States and Canada. *Clin Pediatr*. 2004; **43**(8): 729–35.

Lane J, Gottlieb R. Improving the interviewing and self-assessment skills of medical students: is it time to readopt videotaping as an educational tool? *Ambul Pediatr*. 2004; **4**(3): 244–8.

Lane L, Gottlieb R. Structured clinical observations: a method to teach clinical skills with limited time and financial resources. *Pediatr*. 2000; **105**(4): 973–7.

4

Feedback and Evaluation

Len Kelly

Feedback and evaluation are very connected conceptually. Feedback is the key component of formative evaluation and delineates the gap between where the learner is presently, and their preferred level of performance. Good feedback helps the learner diminish that gap.

Evaluation is generally considered "formative" when it involves "informing" or "forming" the student into a more accomplished clinician. We do this with our day-to-day interactions as we direct and give feedback. While we might like to "form" them into our own likeness, but thankfully human diversity intercedes. Like all aspects of medical education, formative evaluation in a clinical setting always begins at patient safety and winds its way through rotation objectives and should be served up with some encouragement.

Many medical education programs are developing required formative assessments in the form of documented, observed learner–patient interactions. These constitute formative evaluation as their purpose is to help the development of the learner, even though there may be a scoring system added to the document supplied by the program. This reflects educational rigor and is also consistent with movement toward "competency-based" evaluation. It is not enough to document that the learner sees a certain number of cases and clinical scenarios. Educational programs need to ensure the learners are competent and that requires clinical teachers, including community-based preceptors, to see learner performance with their own eyes. This takes practice, skill and some time.

When evaluation is documented and judged against an expected standard as we do in the end of rotation assessment forms, this is summative evaluation. This assessment summarizes and adds-up (summates) the learner's progress, achievement of objectives and ranking against benchmarks established by the program. Summative evaluations forms are legal documents. They are vetted by the academic program and are subject to institutional appeal and even legal proceedings in the case of a disputed assessment. What a teacher writes, therefore, must be accurate, objective, defensible and yes, legible!

GIVING FEEDBACK

Giving feedback is often avoided by both the clinical teacher and the learner. Why is that? It involves a new aspect of the teacher–learner relationship that might be challenging and requires dealing with unknowns and negatives. We may also be concerned that it will upset the good working relationship we are developing with the learner. It may be that this is a new educational exercise for the preceptor and they really do not know how to do it well! We may be unskilled ourselves in receiving feedback both cognitively and emotionally. Teachers may have received negative feedback during their own medical training and it remains an enduring memory for them. They have never been given a practical or theoretical framework on how to proceed. This may feel like the medical educational equivalent of "delivering bad news."

Suffice to say, it is typically a challenging skill and practicing it more often will both normalize it and improve our performance. Many of us think of feedback as a time of judgment, a time when we tell the learner what they are doing wrong. In fact, the educational literature stresses removing judgment from the process. That may mean that in reality the practice will lie somewhere between the two. Some authors admit that preceptor judgment is required in giving feedback, particularly if we must point out deficiencies which the student has omitted from their own self-assessment. Ideally, we are facilitating the learner discovering their strengths and weaknesses.

Feedback is about giving information to a learner in a safe and useful manner (*see* Figure 4.1). It must include: respect, honesty and accuracy. As clinical teachers, we need to develop a simple formulaic way of proceeding (*see* Table 4.1). That way we can reproduce it often in a credible manner without much stress.

Table 4.1 Feedback Essentials

Good feedback:
➤ includes being descriptive rather than judgmental
➤ supports learner's self-esteem
➤ is planned and organized
➤ actively involves the learner's thoughts and feelings
➤ is behavior specific

Poor feedback:
➤ is unpredictable
➤ demoralizes
➤ is judgmental
➤ generalizes, positively or negatively
➤ does not focus on specific behaviors or decisions
➤ does not elicit the thoughts or feelings of the learner

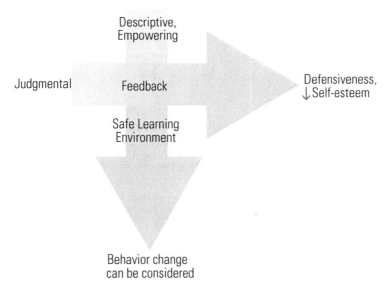

Figure 4.1 Safe Learning Environment

Theories of Educational Feedback

The classic "feedback sandwich" might do in a pinch, but you may find that you are able to do better. Simply put, the feedback sandwich is an Oreo cookie with mustard in the middle: give a positive statement before and after a negative one. Learners will know that criticism follows praise and may learn to cringe at both.

The more established Pendleton's rules, first published in 1984, have become a conventional medical education method and contain many good features.

Following Pendleton's process, the *learner speaks first* and describes what they *did well*; that is re-enforced and discussed with the teacher.

The process is repeated with a self-assessment by the learner of what *could have been done better*, again followed by reinforcement by the facilitator and a discussion of what skills or approach might work better.

The critical benefit of these rules is two-fold: the learner goes first with their self-assessment and both strengths and weaknesses are addressed.

In the 1990s Silverman further developed feedback theory with a framework which was called "agenda-led, outcome-based analysis" (ALBOA). In short, the learner sets the agenda by identifying any problem-spots in the interview they have just conducted. Together with the preceptor, they troubleshoot what approach or skill development is required. Simultaneously, the clinical teacher acknowledges what the student has done well. The refining of interviewing skill options can even be rehearsed by some role-playing on the spot. One of the keys of this method is creating a supportive environment in which to suggest alternate approaches the learner might try. It differs from Peterson's method in being more learner-focused than approach-driven. You begin where the learner has identified they struggled. In both methods, the learner goes first. The ALBOA observation guides are generally referred to as the Calgary–Cambridge Observation Guides and are widely available (*see* Further Reading at the end of this chapter).

Synthesis: Giving Feedback in Dynamic Situations; 'On the Fly'

➤ Let the learner go first. It is uncanny how accurate learners are at self-evaluation. If, for example, they document a difficulty you also perceive, you can agree with them, compliment them on their perceptiveness and move on to the creative problem-solving, which is the easy part.

➤ Be timely. After a difficult clinical scenario in which you and the learner have participated, you need to compose yourself. Then try to save some energy for the learner: How do you feel? Are you OK? Do you have any questions about this difficult patient scenario or outcome? At the very least, discuss it the next day. If the incident is not a serious clinical incident, but does include something you would like to feedback to the learner, do not store it for future reference. Deal with it that day. It is unfair to "bring up dirty laundry" days or weeks later, or in a summative evaluation if they have not been dealt with at the time. The learner needs to be able to explain themselves. They also need to learn from teaching moments when they occur, so their memory is accurate and the experience fresh.

➤ Be specific. Telling someone they seem bored, or otherwise exhibited what you perceive as a poor attitude does not facilitate much learning and is quite subjective. Clinicians may accurately diagnose a certain attitude, but that does not mean the learner will be so perceptive or even be in agreement. One must refer to specific behaviors or comments made by the learner. During observation, quoting back to the learner their exact phrases is often eye-opening. "Did I really say that?" Or the teacher can ask if the student sees how that question or comment might be perceived as judgmental/critical by the patient? This is quite different from saying you felt the learner was judgmental or rude, which will likely illicit a defensive response.

➤ Say something positive. False compliments are not the order of the day, but there really is need for some encouragement for learners, particularly those who are struggling.

➤ Keep the amount of feedback to small digestible amounts in the middle of a busy day, so that you can both move forward with patient care.

Scheduled Feedback Sessions

I use a combination of the above theories. I believe the learning environment is one of the key first steps (*see* Figure 4.2). I acknowledge that this observation–feedback process is stressful for the learner. I make it clear how the session will go and how the learner will complete the patient care before any feedback takes place.

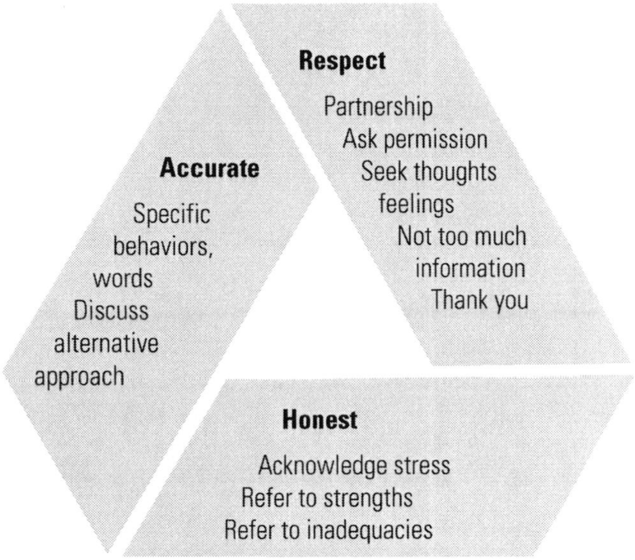

Respect

Partnership
Ask permission
Seek thoughts
feelings
Not too much
information
Thank you

Accurate

Specific
behaviors,
words
Discuss
alternative
approach

Honest

Acknowledge stress
Refer to strengths
Refer to inadequacies

Figure 4.2 Feedback Overview

I generally schedule these observation and feedback sessions toward the end of the day, so that the learner will have some free time coming up and time to regroup, and even reflect, if it has been challenging for them.

When the learner has come out of the patient care session for which they will receive feedback, I give them some breathing room (*see* Table 4.2). They literally may need to take a deep breath to allow them to change gears from nervously giving patient care to now being asked for self-evaluation.

"How was that?"
"How did that feel for you?"

Then into specific parts of the interaction:

"What went well for you?"
"What was challenging for you?"

I facilitate by agreeing with accurate self-assessment. For things that went well:

"I agree that worked well"

For awkward moments with the patient:

"When you said these words (recount verbatim from your notes) what were you trying to achieve? Did it work? What effect might it have on a patient? What effect did it appear to have on this patient?"

Problem solving:

"What might have worked better? Are there opportunities for developing this skill?"

Open agenda:

"Anything else you experienced or would like to add?"

Thanks:

"Thanks for the energy and attention you have put into this self-assessment session."

Document the session briefly in "field" notes which can be included in the learner's file. These are short descriptions of the presenting problem, how the learner did and any identified areas for improvement.

Table 4.2 Overview of Essentials of Feedback

1	Debrief
2	Learner goes first:
	What went well?
	What did not?
3	How to improve
4	Teacher references specific observed words or behaviors
5	Thanks

Feedback on Videotapes

It is important to both protect the student from too much negative information and respect their learning autonomy. If videotaping has been used as a monitoring method, patient confidentiality and consent also need to be protected. This is especially true if the tape will be viewed by other students and teachers. When giving feedback on videotaped interviews, the student should control the play and stop functions of the tape. Using the agenda-based approach, the student begins and comments on areas of the tape they have found problematic. To do this, the student may need to have the time and opportunity to preview the tape on their own. If the feedback is being done with a small group of students (ideally fewer than four), it is best if other students are permitted to comment solely on what their colleague has done well. House rules should define that the facilitator is the only person, other than the student-interviewer, who may point out deficits. Otherwise, the learner will hear too much (repetitive) negative feedback. If all learners are going to present tapes, the process is repeated. Upon completion of each of their debriefs, the facilitator then has a composite list of types of things which all the students have identified which need to be improved. There will usually be concordance of problem areas across all of the interviews. Mediating strategies can be individually or jointly explored and even reinforced with some role-playing. The final step is to set goals which learners can try to implement in future settings on the areas they have identified.

Multi-source Input into Learner Feedback/Evaluation

If you work in a group practice, you must ensure that the learner spends enough time with one or two teachers so that they may have a grounded opinion when evaluation time arrives. It is helpful to discuss the learners at clinic meetings to obtain an overview of how the learner is doing. This also helps to point out behavior patterns that might not otherwise be noticed. I have, at times, made a transparency of the evaluation form and gone over what the group might place as ranking and comments. More importantly, documenting successful and unsuccessful behaviors can be accomplished. Stating that a particular student is "doing fine" is not going to be enough documentation at evaluation time.

Another opportunity for input to judge the learner's performance is to check with the other health professionals (nurses, occupational therapists (OTs) physiotherapists (PTs)) and the office support staff. Learners who ingratiate themselves to their clinical preceptor, yet treat others poorly, are demonstrating unprofessional behavior and this must be addressed. Remember to ensure specific interactions are documented of what was both said and done if any feedback is to be given. General judgmental comments do not help and cannot be passed on to the learner.

Seek Feedback Yourself

Clearly there is a power imbalance between the learner and the clinical teacher. The learner may not want to share any negative thoughts about your teaching. The program will have them complete a confidential evaluation form of their learning experience after the rotation and, at some point that will be fed back to you. I do find that asking indirectly: "Are there any things we might consider changing before the next student arrives?" may elicit some helpful feedback. I tell learners that we are always trying to improve the learning experience and any advice they may have would be helpful. But you can only take this so far. The learner is primarily invested in getting a reasonable evaluation and disputing a poor evaluation if necessary.

Be Consistent

Develop a systematic approach to formative assessment. Create a learning environment. For effective feedback, let the learner go first. Remember it is about information sharing, not judging. Always find something positive. Be specific. Document. It is probably one of the more challenging tasks we have as teachers and takes some time, skill and practice to become reasonable at it.

EVALUATION

We have seen that formative assessment in the form of direct observation and feedback needs to be timely, specific, supportive and non-judgmental. Ideally, it fosters learning. Summative evaluation compares the learner with an established competency benchmark and essentially with their peers (*see* Figure 4.3). Earlier formative evaluation should mimic the summative process in a supportive way. The feedback the learner has received will help them acquire physical exam and communication skills which will be tested by program-defined OSCEs or SOOs. Medical knowledge discussions which have occurred throughout the rotation during end-of-day case reviews or case management chats identify weaker areas of knowledge. These will be tested in future multiple-choice exams.

The summative evaluation encountered by all community-based preceptors is typically the end of rotation form. If no formative work has occurred, then these sessions are abrupt hallmarks. This is not uncommon. They become "high-stakes feedback" occasions rather than significant junctions in an ongoing evaluative process. In a perfect world, the summative evaluation should contain few surprises if the formative work has been done and documented.

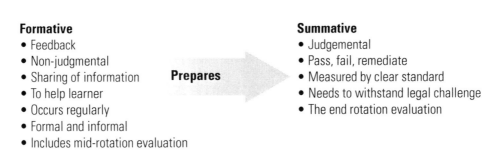

Formative
- Feedback
- Non-judgmental
- Sharing of information   **Prepares**
- To help learner
- Occurs regularly
- Formal and informal
- Includes mid-rotation evaluation

Summative
- Judgemental
- Pass, fail, remediate
- Measured by clear standard
- Needs to withstand legal challenge
- The end rotation evaluation

Figure 4.3 Formative and Summative Evaluation

Program-specific summative evaluation needs to accomplish two things. The first is to identify sub-standard performances and weed out inappropriate candidates for the profession. To achieve this, the process must be able to resist legal challenges which will often rely on competent and consistent documentation throughout the rotation. The second function of summative evaluations is actually formative: they document improvement and give the learner feedback on areas that need more attention. This information may be useful in career choices for the learner and the planning of subsequent elective rotations. Even the high-achiever should receive some useful information from a proper evaluation.

ROLE OF CLINICAL TEACHER

We might often feel like distant cogs in the academic wheel, but our role in evaluation is critical. We are the preceptors most likely to have observed the learner in real-life patient situations. We are in the best position to judge if they are safe and acceptable to progress to the next level. What we know from the education literature is that multiple sources of evaluation, on multiple occasions, will likely give us the most accurate assessment. Clinical teachers are the experts in the field. We can give a specific but also holistic, impression of the candidate.

A landmark paper by Van der Vleuten in 2010 reflected on the importance of the holistic assessment. Despite being able to check off all the tick boxes on an evaluation, the clinical supervisor may still have an unquiet feeling that the learner is not ready to move forward. While highly subjective, this assessment is also highly informed and quite valuable. Objective measures of communication skills such as OSCEs may in fact tell us more about ourselves, the question-writers, than the communication skills of the learner. The scoring is objective but may not always validly portray all one would like to know about a learner. Van der Vleuten's article pushes the boundaries of assessment and validates the importance of the subjective aspect of assessment.

So, our sense of whether the learner is safe to proceed, our "gut" intuition, is an important barometer. The challenge community-based preceptors face is how to creatively include that in the program assessment for the benefit of both the learner and the profession.

A FAILING EVALUATION

Failing evaluations are very uncommon, but constitute a critical teaching event for the preceptor. Two things commonly occur. The first is that the preceptor will assume they are to blame. Perhaps they are misjudging the learner? Could they have done more to help the learner along? The second thing is that the problem is often evident very early on in the rotation. Management of the difficult learner will be discussed in Chapter 8, but here it is important to point out the need to get teaching support and document issues early. As we know, any documentation and feedback must be specific and timely. A poor evaluation may eventually be legally challenged. It withstands such a challenge if it is preceded by a paper trail documenting feedback, discussions and educational consultations. Discuss the issues with teaching colleagues and contact your program support person. Typically, it is the program director who may have intervention strategies to suggest and who may have encountered previous problems with this learner or similar issues with other learners.

Bear in mind that a pass on the mid-term evaluation may be legally inconsistent with a failed end-of-rotation grade. So address the issue early, and if the learner is heading toward a poor final assessment, it also needs to be documented on the official mid-rotation paperwork. This is distressing for both parties. Bear in mind also that, as a preceptor, you do not have the ultimate say in how the program will deal with the learner. Your input is into the particular rotation performance and behavior alone.

Appeal Process

Be somewhat familiar with the appeal process of your program so that you can direct the learner appropriately if they disagree with you. Any appeal will hinge on how much observation, feedback and documentation has occurred. If the student has passed the mid-term evaluation, failing them on the final one will be a hard sell to the challengers of your process. Keep that in mind, when you are half-way through the rotation with a difficult learner.

Store your Field Notes/Evaluations

Keep a file of all your field notes and evaluations. Years later, a student may want a reference for applying to another program. After several years of teaching, you may recognize many ex-students at a conference or another academic gathering, but not well enough to put any useful information down in a helpful reference letter for them. If you have a filing system on evaluations, you can go back and see when the student was with your practice, how long they were there and specifics about their capabilities. This also gives you a back-up copy at the time of the evaluation if it gets lost in travel to the program. I have had to go back years when a previous student required a reference for entering a Master's program after several years in their clinical practice. If your program has converted to electronic evaluations, still keep an independent copy for your own reference.

SUMMARY

Feedback and evaluation are the most stressful parts of the community-based medical education dialectic. Preceptors are not alone in feeling somewhat inadequate in these areas and would be well served to seek out faculty development sessions that deal with these issues.

FURTHER READING
Feedback

Archer J. State of the science in health professional education: effective feedback. *Med Educ.* 2010; 44: 101–8.

Chodhury R, Kalu G. Learning to give feedback in medical education. *Obstet Gynecol.* 2004; **6**: 243–7.

Delima TJ, Arnold R. Giving feedback. *J Palliat Med.* 2011; **14**(2): 233–9.

Ende J. Feedback in clinical medical education. *JAMA.* 1998; **250**: 777–81.

Gigante J, Dell M, Sharkey A. Getting beyond "good job": how to give effective feedback. *Pediatr.* 2011; **27**: 205–7.

Hewson M, Little M. Giving feedback in medical education. *JGIM.* 1998; **13**: 111–16.

O'Brien M, Oxman A, Davis D, *et al.* Audit and feedback: effects of professional practice and healthcare outcomes: *Cochrane Database Syst Rev.* 2003; **3**: CD000259.

Pendleton D, Schonfield T, Tate P, *et al. The Consultation: an approach to learning and teaching.* Oxford: Oxford University Press; 1984.

Pendleton D, Schonfield, Tate T, *et al.* Learning and teaching about the consultation. In: *The New Consultation: developing doctor–patient communication.* Oxford: Oxford University Press; 2003.

Silverman J, Kurtz S, Draper J. *Agenda-led Outcome-based Analysis.* Available at: www.gp-training.net/training/communication_skills/calgary (accessed August 9, 2011)

Veloski J, Boex J, Grasberger M, *et al.* Systematic review of the literature on assessment, feedback and physicians' clinical performance? BBME Guide No. 7. *Med Teach.* 2006; **28**(2): 117–28.

Evaluation

Epstein R. Assessment in medical education. *N Engl J Med.* 2007; **356**(4): 387–96.

Freidman B, Snadden D, Hesketh A. Linking appraisal of PRHO professional competence of junior doctors to their education. *Med Teach.* 2004; **26**(1): 63–70.

Hatem C, Searle N, Gunderman R, *et al.* The educational attribute and responsibilities of effective medical educators. *Acad Med.* 2011; **86**(4): 474–80.

Holmbe E, Sherbino J, Long D, *et al.* The role of assessment in competency-based medical education. *Med Teach.* 2010; **32**: 676–82.

Kilminister S, Jolly B. Effective supervision in clinical practice settings; a literature review. *Med Educ.* 2000; **34**: 827–40.

Rushton A. Formative assessment: a key to deep learning? *Med Teach.* 2005; **27**(6): 509–13.

Stake R. *Standards-based and Responsive Evaluation.* Thousand Oaks, California, Sage; 2004.

Townsend A, Mcilvenny S, Miller C, *et al.* The use of an objective structured clinical examination (OSCE) for formative and summative assessment in a general practice clinical attachment and its relationship to final medical school examination performance. *Med Educ.* 2001; **35**: 841–6.

Van der Vleuten C, Schwirth L, Scheele F, *et al.* The assessment of professional compe tence: building blocks for theory development. *Best Prac Res Clin Obstet Gynecol.* 2010; **24**(6): 703–14.

5

Teaching

Len Kelly

Medical teaching is somewhat like parenting. Our skills are learned by experience when we were learners. In large part, we emulate those who taught us and evolve through our experience and critical teaching moments. Our teaching style generally needs to fit with our personality. Like parenting, we need consistency, fairness and a degree of predictability. There are principles to adult education that we shall touch on, but one need not necessarily be aware of them to be a good teacher.

Clinical teachers are expert clinicians. Primarily, that alludes to our clinical pattern recognition. We instantly perceive a septic or psychotic patient, particularly when it comes to patients we have known for some time. This puts us at a terrific knowledge advantage over the learner. It is important to use this in a positive manner. Discussions of common scenarios, predisposing risk factors and their thinking about diagnosis is fair game. Teaching the learner to read your thoughts and play "What am I thinking" does not develop their independent judgment. Our learners do not need to arrive at the same endpoint/diagnosis as an experienced clinical teacher, but they need to develop tools to reach a reasonable endpoint. Learners recognize this. They spend a lot of energy trying to learn how we do what we do. How do we think or approach a given problem? I tell students that neither of us will know everything, but we may need to develop an approach. Learners want to learn our critical clinical thinking and it is of real educational advantage for them when we share our thinking process with them (*see* Table 5.1). For the preceptor, much of this is unconscious and sharing it with a learner will require some reflection to understand how to make it explicit. This chapter will look at many of these issues in some depth and give some educational background to many sound teaching practices.

Table 5.1 Ingredients in the Teaching Dyad

Preceptors need to be:	
	supportive
	curious
	accessible
Students need to:	
	work hard
	keep the spark
	be part of the team

CORRIDOR CONSULTATION

Listen

The quick corridor consultation is an important microcosm of the teaching relationship. Preceptors need to recognize and honor this (*see* Table 5.2). For the purpose of this discussion, we will assume the learner is a postgraduate resident, as undergraduates will already have close supervision. When the resident or junior doctor stops you between exam rooms – literally in the corridor – or comes to your office with a question, they need your undivided attention. Put down what you are doing, turn to them and listen. If we role-model good listening to the learner, they may realize the skill is also useful to them with patients. Giving them the time they need, even if you do not have any, honors the barriers they have overcome to speak to you, such as:

> "My question is not important"
> "I should know what to do"
> "My preceptor is too busy to interrupt"

By listening, we are telling the learner that we want them to ask questions when they are uncertain about something. It also recognizes that they are having a difficult time with something, or might be stressed by something and that is normal for a learner. The patient they are seeing could be very ill or makes them worried or uncomfortable. Consider that the learner may be about to make a mistake and they are checking with you before doing so!

Clarify Agenda

Let the resident tell you their concern, even in simple terms. If they are completely overwhelmed by the scenario and want you to come and rescue them – do so. But first ascertain what has gotten them so off-balance: an angry patient, a learner insecurity? If they are still in control of the patient–doctor consultation, clarify specifically what it is they need help with: communication, diagnosis or treatment plan? This reinforces their developing autonomy and helps you to understand at what level you need to participate. It may be something simple. It just takes a second to ask the resident specifically what they want help with: something specific or everything. Either is acceptable, but they tell you very different things about how the learner is doing.

Respond and Facilitate Learning

After meeting the patient and helping overcome the roadblock the resident encountered, facilitate the learner taking back the consultation. Do not completely take over if the learner only needed a small nudge or diagnostic advice. Check if they can take it to an appropriate conclusion before leaving, so that they will not have to come and get you again for the same patient. We respect the learner's autonomy by playing the role they have requested of us and no more. A modest aliquot of "pearls" will often suffice. A supportive learning environment is established: it is all right to ask for help, and the learner can still retain some control.

Encourage Asking

At the end of the day, point out that you appreciated them asking for help when they did. I specifically tell them that the learner who concerns me most is the one who feels uncomfortable about something and does not seek advice. They need to know that you will be there when they are concerned, or out of their depth with a patient, and that it is not acceptable to err in silence because you seem too busy to interrupt. This also helps the resident to "listen-to-their-gut" and seek help appropriately – a career-long process.

Table 5.2 Corridor Consultation

➤ Listen attentively
➤ Agree on agenda
➤ Respond to request
➤ Facilitate learning
➤ Encourage asking

AMBULATORY CARE
Graded Responsibility and Clinical Supervision

Undergraduate students' levels of competence and learning objectives require different supervision strategies than postgraduate residents (*see* Table 5.3). This is intuitive and is easily operationalized. Both types of learners will need a similar initial orientation, most easily described as "puppy-dogging."

Puppy-dogging

The fresh keenness of the novice learner is what keeps many of us interested in teaching. When a learner first arrives in our practice, they accompany us in to see patients that we are booked to see. I introduce the learner to the patient and then delve into what the presenting concern is. An intuitive preceptor will gain a sense of how much of this passive exposure a learner needs. Usually an hour or two is sufficient. A particularly nervous or awkward student may need to do this for a day or so, but this would be unusual. This "introductory offer" is sufficient to let the learner see the practice style we employ and how the pace of the office optimally occurs. After several hours of this, the senior learner can be sent off on their own to see their booked patients. The junior learner will continue to see the preceptor's patients, most often going in to see them alone first. The teacher then returns to the student and patient and goes over the history and findings to ensure completeness. They jointly take the consultation to completion. This style will continue for the junior learner over the duration of the rotation, while the senior learner has moved down the hall a bit to function more autonomously.

Table 5.3 Graded Levels of Responsibility and Supervision

Undergraduate Learner
- ➤ Every patient also seen by teacher
- ➤ Cases discussed during patient flow
- ➤ End-of-day debriefing
- ➤ End-of-day focused chart review

Postgraduate Learner
- ➤ Sees patients independently
- ➤ Has immediate access to supervisor
- ➤ Corridor consultations during clinic
- ➤ Thorough chart review daily

Undergraduate Learners

Many learners are more focused on the preceptor than the patient, as a result of the educational power differential. We need to create a supportive learning environment to decrease the learner's stress – but also to gently focus them on the patient. We may need to encourage patient-centered thinking.

> "How was the patient today?"
> "Why do you think they came in today?"
> "How does the patient feel about all of this?"

By asking these common-sense questions, we are giving a balance to the often train-like series of closed-ended questions that learners are beginning to develop around history of present illness, review of symptoms, etc. Additionally, learners are faced with two competing clinical agendas: being thorough and being problem-focused. For a busy preceptor, that can mean the difference between "taking too long" and "getting to the point." This is particularly true of learners who have just finished a hospital-based rotation or a specialty rotation where one-hour long consultations are common. We need to explicitly re-orient the student to be problem-focused and timely in their assessment. During problem-focused consultations experienced clinical teachers intuitively know how wide to cast the net. The novice will often not grasp this skill yet and will need gentle re-orienting. The exception to this is the patient in the office for whom the wheels have fallen off – they need a lot of our time and our students' time. Additionally, hospital admissions and annual health exams require thorough exams including complete history and physicals. Having the capacity to do complete multi-system exams is a valuable skill to have. Ambulatory care often keeps it in reserve for cases that require it.

An interesting finding with undergraduate students is their definite comfort with extensive history taking and discomfort with diagnosis or treatment plan. When I ask them what they think is wrong, most students will answer by reciting more history. That pattern will repeat itself. It is uncanny how often this occurs, as illogical as it seems. I persist in asking for some approach to diagnosis. It is fair to reinforce with most undergraduates that they can avoid Latin words or "medicalese" if that is a barrier. Telling me the patient has "a stomach problem" can be a reasonable starting point, particularly if they are nervous. I then acknowledge that "diagnosis" and ask simple questions:

> "Do you think it is something serious?"
> "Do we need to do any investigations?"
> "Do you think they need any treatment?"

These are baby steps, but as the famous coach, Vince Lombardi pointed out, "you can only go as fast as your slowest learner." We are establishing a safe environment by simplifying some of the language and knowledge hurdles. More importantly, we are acknowledging and modeling the importance of clinical reasoning. The complaint may, or may not, relate to a "diagnosis," which may, or may not, be amenable to treatment. It also reinforces that we can still be supportive and listen to the patient, regardless of how well we score on the "medical detective scale." Undergraduates need to be slowly and safely led from the comfortable forests of history taking, onto the more dangerous hunting plains of diagnosis.

Undergraduates often have a reasonable level of clinical skills by the time they are in a community-based rotation, but this is an important time for students to consolidate simple skills they will perform throughout their career. Make sure they are doing them correctly.

Their learning benefits from settling on a relevant topic daily, around which the student can spend some time reading for review the following day. Applied knowledge will predictably be "spotty" in many undergraduates. Basic standard topics would include hypertension, diabetes and pregnancy. Or, choose a particular drug or class of drug for discussion. The objective is that the learner associates reading around patients and their care, which is a career-long enterprise.

CONFIDENCE AND COMPETENCE IN LONGITUDINAL CLINICAL CLERKSHIPS

Longitudinal clinical clerkships in community-based settings give the student the advantage of learning in a familiar setting, even as they go through different, and often concurrent, rotations. This also gives their clinical teachers an overview of their progress as well as difficult times. While every student is unique, Walters, an Australian medical educator, has noted a somewhat predictable flow of confidence that can occur during clerkship, to which I have added a competence gradient (*see* Figure 5.1). This may occur in urban tertiary care rotations as well, but seems more noticeable in a community-based setting.

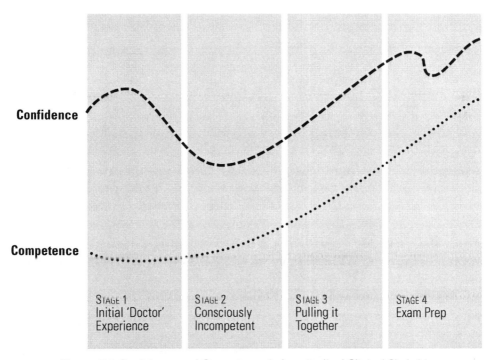

Figure 5.1 Confidence and Competence in Longitudinal Clinical Clerkship

Stage 1 gives the student their initial experience of "being a doctor." They wore a white coat, spoke to a patient and went on hospital rounds for the first time!

Later, they did their first suturing. There is a lot of appropriate excitement in this honeymoon period, with a lot of "initial" confidence and a beginner's level of competence.

In Stage 2, the clerk experiences their limitations in knowledge and skills. The generic approach they used initially lets them down; perhaps they encounter challenging patients. They have to learn additional knowledge and approaches. Despite this unpleasant experience (what translational learning theorists call a "disorienting dilemma"), it causes a broadening of their learning and contributes to their competence. They may express their disheartenment to their preceptor. This allows us to put it in a positive perspective as a part of the learning process.

Stage 3 is pulling it all together and applying more functional approaches and additional knowledge. They are developing some rudimentary clinical reasoning; distinguishing "sick" from "not sick;" changing their history and examination scripts in response to patient cues and beginning to get on the same wavelength as their preceptors.

Stage 4 is time to prepare for exams. Hitting the books again complements their clinical experience and allows for incorporation of previous pathophysiology knowledge (sometimes called integration or elaboration of knowledge in educational literature). Confidence waxes and wanes with exam anxiety but, generally, competence is enhanced.

Postgraduate Learners

Orientation

Residents or junior registrars bring out a more mature and reflective level of discussion around patient care. It takes several days for the mature learner to hit their stride and find a flow to the clinical day. They are learning the office system, trying to remember staff members' names, care for patients and figure out the investigation and referral threshold for a given preceptor. This is a tall order, and it is reassuring to see the resident asking for help with this a lot, during the first few days. It is wise to let them know that you expect that they will not know how things are done in this practice location and that you welcome inquiries.

Uncertainty

Postgraduate learners may be used to undertaking more specialist referrals as this was the norm in the urban centers where they trained. They may need to be informed about the visiting specialist schedule or the challenge long-distance referrals make for your patients and their families. If the postgraduates share one tendency, it might be to over-investigate. Their comfort level with uncertainty is just developing and they have been exposed to the latest technology in their earlier urban hospital-based rotations. It is our task to point out explicitly and by role-modeling that clinical uncertainty is common and often a part of the on-going patient–doctor relationship. A wizened colleague used to remark: "That was the worst case of whatever it was, I have ever seen!"

COMMUNICATION

Another common resident issue is their comfort in using predominantly closed-ended questions and a lack of expertise with open-ended ones. This is analogous to the undergraduate student's comfort with history taking. Uncertainty is just becoming a part of the mature learner's day. Observed patient interviews will commonly demonstrate that the resident departs from open-ended questions before they really understand why the patient is there. They then efficiently travel a route to a dead end and have to start all over again. When you observe a resident interview, count the number of open-ended questions they ask. There may be one or two. They are uncomfortable asking any more, even though open-ended questions are the key starting point which gives direction to subsequent questioning. They need to be encouraged to hang in there, and repeatedly go back to the patient with open-ended queries until they see some light to follow. In this way, they are no different than the rest of us, although for the experienced clinician, it may reflect impatience as well as discomfort with uncertainty. Clinicians often wait less than 20 seconds before interrupting a patient who is trying to tell them why they are there in their own way. Investing in silence and open-ended questions at the beginning of an interview is a worthwhile endeavor, partly because it is respectful listening, but also because we may find out a lot more about the patient's issue.

Time Management

At first glance, it may seem odd to include a section on time management in a chapter on teaching. However, postgraduate resident learners, almost universally, struggle with this issue and frequently it is in the transition from previous hospital-based consulting service rotations to a community setting that time management problems become apparent. Time management is an important practical aptitude for residents to acquire to survive in the real world. Effective management of one's clinical time can have a significant impact on personal and professional satisfaction and impacts on patient care (*see* Table 5.4).

Patients who are not seen at their scheduled time feel less valued by their clinician and a learner who does not use time effectively can negatively impact patient flow in a clinic. This reduces the educational opportunities for interaction with the preceptor as they both struggle to deal with the backlog.

Time management also indirectly speaks to a learner's interview and communication competence. Learners are exposed to an emphasis on communication and diagnostic issues throughout their training, and community-based practices may be the first opportunity they encounter to effectively manage their time. Given practical limitations placed upon clinicians, quality communication is more highly valued than quantity. Learners may have the impression that spending more time with a patient is better quality care. Cape's 2002 study of 176 general practice patients found that there was no association with actual interview time and patient satisfaction, but rather with "perceived" time spent. He postulated that patients experience the quality of the time they spend with their physician more than the quantity. Dugdale's 1999 and 2008 reviews recommended the most productive intervention for time management was likely to be improved physician communication skill. This was most effectively accomplished by: rapport building, up-front agenda setting and responding to patient emotional cues appropriately.

Learners need direction in establishing a comfortable setting for patients: how they introduce themselves and setting the agreed clinical agenda for the interview. It is also effective to take notes during the interview if it does not interfere with communication – though most residents need to listen more and write less. Terminating an interview when the time has elapsed may need focused attention for the learner, and the preceptor can pass on their ways of achieving this. Judicious use of follow-up appointments with set agendas are often something the resident needs help incorporating into their management. So time management is a key learning opportunity in a community-based practice. Preceptors need to let the learner know how they are booked and set an initial slow pace. Office staff and preceptors can help the resident accomplish effective care that will include practical interview issues, with a focus on quality communication.

Table 5.4 Time Management Essentials

➤ Listen to patient vs delivering "educational" monologues
➤ Quality time vs actual time
➤ Set interview agenda early
➤ Good time management = respect for patient, staff, self/family
➤ Minimize interruptions
➤ Have verbal strategies for ending interviews

PATIENT CONTEXT

Once these practicalities have taken on a predictable pattern and the resident seems to have a handle on the patient care, it is worth exploring some of the patient's previous health challenges and how they may have contributed to where they are now. It is also worth asking reflective questions about why this patient presents in this way, at this time. We take for granted that the patient has phoned for an appointment, sat in the waiting room and waited for their name to be called. But what is that like for a severely anxious patient or one without a phone? It is useful to explore with the resident what the patient's experience is like beyond the office confines. We need to encourage them to listen well to patients and deepen that listening when necessary.

THE LEARNER WHO DOES NOT "FIT IN"

The learner who does not fit in will attract a lot more of your attention. They require more feedback and certainly greater attention to documentation during their rotation. This learner may be from another culture, they may just be quirky or they may not be suitable for a career in medicine. A specific focus on behavior, rather than our perception of attitude, will need to be documented. Seek advice early from colleagues as well as the program director if the student seems well below par or unsafe. A robust discussion on this topic takes place in Chapter 8 on the problem and difficult learner.

CHART REVIEW

Going over charts at the end of the day with a senior learner is a basic standard for supervising residents. It acknowledges the clinical teacher is responsible for the patient's care and should be our minimal standard for supervising postgraduate learners – in addition to regular direct observation. Postgraduate learners typically have an educational license and the patients have been booked to see them. The flow of patients is initially reasonably slow to give the learner time to become used to the operation of the clinic, to consolidate their thinking and have time to ask for help while the patient is still in the clinic. Any patient not discussed, or seen by the preceptor during the course of the day, needs to be reviewed at the end of the day. This gives an opportunity to check on the appropriateness of diagnosis and management.

About one hour needs to be set aside. The learner gives a brief synopsis of each patient's presenting complaint, other issues and the treatment and follow-up plan. Allow the learner to handle the chart, as they will need to take a quick glance to remember the patient and their interaction and treatment. They then hand it over to you for assessment of the clarity of the written note and your signature or initial. As cases are discussed, topics for further study or discussion are identified. Cases in which care has gone awry necessitate the resident calling the patient directly by phone or arranging urgent follow-up. If the learner has been given the appropriate training, degree of responsibility and access to their supervisor throughout the day, this actually occurs quite rarely. In our practice, the teacher signs off each note to acknowledge they have discussed the patient care and agree. This ensures that learners are not taken advantage of by the teacher benefiting from billings generated by their efforts, but performing little supervision or chart review.

Such daily chart reviews are excellent learning opportunities for both learner and teacher. The senior learner may have just left a specialty rotation and is a bit more up-to-date than their teacher. The teacher can probe, both the clinical thinking from which the management plan arises, as well as particulars such as which medication was used. Even the sharpest senior learner can learn some of the art of medicine, knowledge of the patient over time, previous pertinent life events which can all inform the complete picture of why this patient arrived on this day, with this concern. Chart reviews as the sole day-to-day clinical supervision method are appropriate only for learners at the independent end of the graded responsibility scale. But even these advanced learners will need occasional scheduled direct observation. Junior learners will need closer supervision and the patient will need to be seen before they are discharged. Focused chart reviews are also useful for undergraduate learners, but as all patients have been seen by the student and the preceptor during the clinic, either one of them may choose cases worth discussing.

TEACHING COMMUNICATION SKILLS

Communication skills are a part of the basic skills set of any clinician. Clear empathetic communication is an appropriate expectation of our patients and of our regulatory colleges. In 2007, Tamblyn *et al* found an association between poor scores on communication items in Canadian provincial licensing exams and subsequent medico-legal complaints within a 10-year period. There was a linear relationship, with the lowest quartile scores being most associated with patient complaints. This is quite sobering.

Community-based preceptors may assume that the curriculum has already done some basic communication training before the student arrives in their practice. While that may often be true, we will be involved in assessing those skills in our practice. We therefore need to know how to do this type of assessment, and facilitate the remediation of any deficits our students may have. How do we do this?

In a unique and interesting Swiss study in 2009, by Perron *et al* performed focus groups of 19 internal medicine residency preceptors. They found that participants felt unprepared for taking on a teaching role in communication skills. They felt they did not have the skills and struggled with the time required for this. They thought that faculty development in this area would need to be two-fold: they would have to examine their own communication skills and learn appropriate teaching skills. They were concerned that a teacher's self-esteem was at risk in having their own communication style scrutinized, and recommended external examiners who were not a part of their everyday hierarchy.

This was the first article in the literature which actually categorized how preceptors described the role they played in supervising communication skills. They most commonly became involved after a difficult situation had already occurred, as a "rescuer." The second role was that of a "supporter" who stood by the resident when they anticipated a difficult communication scenario. The third role, described by only a few preceptors, was that of a "clinical teacher." These preceptors facilitated communication improvement in their residents by learning where they ran into trouble, suggesting alternate strategies, observing and giving feedback. Most preceptors in this study felt they were unprepared to function at this optimal level. That is likely true of many of us as well.

TRAINING

Effective communication skills bring out more information from the patient. This eliciting of information is important in grading the students in simulated office oral examinations. Specific communication skill sessions are best done just before clinical clerkship as the instructional learning is highly reinforced by experiential learning. Often the coursework itself includes experiential components such as role-playing, videotaping and observation. Once clinical clerkship begins, most learning will be experiential: with real patients, simulated patients or role-playing with the preceptor and other learners. Observation and feedback are important components of learning communication skills. If direct observation is being used, jotting down verbatim learner comments and recounting these to them replaces audio- and videotaping.

Preceptors must develop good communication skills themselves if they are to pass them on. If they find it necessary, they might consider finding an organized course away from their typical work venue if they fear exposing their deficits "close to home." Otherwise, they may take the same training as their students.

Passing these skills onto learners will take some preceptor reflecting, observing, feedback and use of some of the available tools. We may then be equipped to help learners in these important teachable moments and ourselves move from being "rescuer" to "clinical facilitator." How can we encourage appropriate communication skills? Initially, we can do this by role-modeling our own communication style with patients and also with learners themselves.

From the medical education research literature, we know that communication skills can be taught. Medical students (and often their preceptors) avoid psychosocial issues in an interview. This may be because they feel unskilled in dealing with the disclosure or it is a countertransference of their own discomfort. This common pattern can be pointed out to the learner. There are teachable strategies developed to address this deficit. Stewart *et al* in 1995, developed the patient-centered paradigm. Using the "FIFE" component of this, one can tease out the psychosocial aspects of the patient–doctor interview:

Function: "How does this affect what you can do?"
Ideas: "What do you think is wrong?"
Feelings: How do you feel about this?"
Expectations: "What were you expecting us to do about this?"

These questions can give our learners, and us, a framework for finding common ground with the patient. Smith's text on patients' stories published in 2001 delivers another acronym (NURS) for clinical empathy:

Name the feeling you sense: "You seem angry about this"
Understand the feeling: "It's understandable you feel this way"
Respect the patient's coping: "You are correct to get this concern discussed"
Support the patient: "We will check into this for you"

INTERVIEWING

One of the hallmarks of patient-centered care is finding common ground. In an interview setting, finding common ground includes defining a place where the patient's agenda and the medical one meet and can be explored. The best time to identify this ground is at the start of the interview. By beginning in an open fashion, both in type of questions, agenda-checking and conversational greeting, we are essentially defining that common ground. We are, perhaps unconsciously, sharing control of the meeting and lessening the power differential that typically exists between physician and patient. Open-ended questions let the patient know that there is room for them to bring their concerns forward. As we proceed into the content of the consultation, we utilize some of our (many) closed-ended questions – but the ground has been defined as having room for the patient to actively participate (*see* Figure 5.2).

During the interview, openings need to be left for the patient to enter the common ground: to ask questions, clarify points or change the focus of discussion. These openings can be pauses or silences to implicitly establish that the patient is still "with us," or explicit checks with overt questions about their understanding.

A shared opening can be the first signal that the common ground is co-defined, that the patients are part-owners of this healthcare "real estate." Checking throughout the interview ensures that this process continues, as does closing the consultation with open-ended, closing questions, such as: "Do you have any questions? Is there anything else? Is this Ok?" and statements indicating that important issues can be re-addressed in the future: "If you think of any questions when you get home we can discuss them on your next visit."

Both the structure and content of the interview need to evoke power-sharing and support patient autonomy. Instructing learners on these predictable

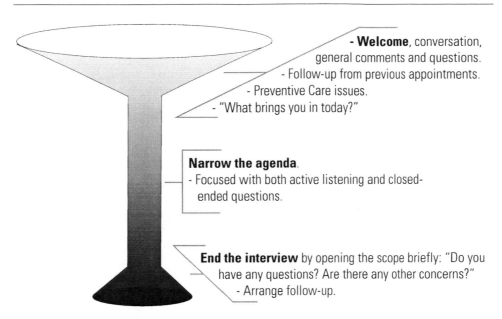

- **Welcome**, conversation, general comments and questions.
- Follow-up from previous appointments.
- Preventive Care issues.
- "What brings you in today?"

Narrow the agenda.
- Focused with both active listening and closed-ended questions.

End the interview by opening the scope briefly: "Do you have any questions? Are there any other concerns?"
- Arrange follow-up.

Figure 5.2 Components of the Patient Interview

parts of a good interview can be instructive for them. Both undergraduate and postgraduate learners tend to be most comfortable with closed-ended questions for disease detection. But even if that is one's sole objective, entering the pattern of closed-ended and disease-specific questions often leads to a dead end. Then the interviewer finds themselves literally back at the beginning. They then choose another "disease script" with its associated predictable questions and it may lead to another dead end. Finally, they are back to the beginning once again! Now, even the most persistent of us may break down and simply ask: "Why are you here today?" By learning this "hard" way, our patients are telling us they will answer as many of our questions they can for us, but that, if we accurately explore early on what their concerns are, things could go quite a bit more efficiently. Time spent in the uncomfortable, uncertainty-filled opening part of healthcare consultations gives us both a shared and accurate agenda.

TEACHING CLINICAL REASONING

Learning clinical reasoning is one of the key "outcomes of choice" of medical education. Interestingly, it is not clear how to help learners get there, partly because it is not clear how we acquired it ourselves. Students want to learn clinical reasoning as that is how their role models function. It is a positive component of the hidden agenda.

A key hallmark of a safe learning environment is the learner's safety in asking questions. Schultz's 2004 survey of 3000 Canadian medical students and residents showed this as the most valued learning attribute. Openness to questions needs to be a fundamental ground rule for a clinical preceptor. There may be a best time and place for lengthy discussions and that can be made clear to the learner, but questions should be welcomed. There are two similar sides to the coin, and both promote learning. Students will learn clinical reasoning by asking us questions, and we can facilitate their learning by asking them questions. In the first instance, we can share what variables went into a given clinical decision we have made. In the second, we can tease from the learner what their thinking is, where their knowledge and intuition may be leading them.

Many medical schools have instituted case-based learning as an initiation to learning the cognitive skills and approach to arrive at a differential diagnosis and move towards treatment. Community-based clinical teachers have the advantage that the patients are real and the questions have clinical significance. This empowers learning. Part of the process is emotional. A survey of 181 graduating Johns Hopkins medical students in 2007–8 by Murinson *et al* found that the highest emotional impact experienced by the students was "finding an exceptional role model." Teaching – or more properly, facilitating – clinical reasoning, requires the preceptor to set up a safe learning environment, so that fear of making mistakes does not interfere with reflective, creative learning. The learner needs to know that they may speak aloud their thoughts, conjectures and worries. Allowing space for this enables them test hypotheses and develop their intuition. This kind of learning needs to be an active process for the learner, so they are engaged.

It can begin simply:

> "Is the patient sick?"
> "Is it serious?"
> "Do you think you know what is wrong with them?"

COGNITIVE STARTING POINTS

We need to understand that the learner and preceptor think very differently about diagnosis and treatment issues (*see* Figure 5.3). The experienced clinical teacher relies increasingly on pattern recognition, which renders them an "expert." Learners are still distinguishing the particular trees, and are quite far from seeing the forest. This is appropriate. With experience, they begin to cluster symptoms as they see which ones we value as significant. Preceptors often need to return to a more measured approach to diagnosis and investigation when they confront a difficult or atypical case. They may even notice that they need to "hit the books" for this patient presentation. When pattern recognition does not supply the diagnosis, they feel lost temporarily, and need to revert to earlier cognitive patterns to cast a wide diagnostic net. The pace of investigation slows and the differential diagnosis remains wide open. This is what it is typically like for most students all the time. With time and explanation, they accumulate some simple patterns that they can recognize. One day, they actually make a diagnosis on their own. These are powerful learning experiences that have been studied very little.

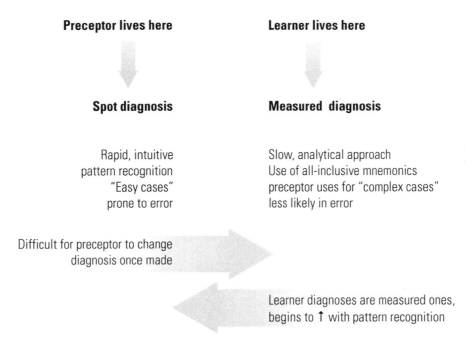

Preceptor lives here

Learner lives here

Spot diagnosis

Measured diagnosis

Rapid, intuitive
pattern recognition
"Easy cases"
prone to error

Slow, analytical approach
Use of all-inclusive mnemonics
preceptor uses for "complex cases"
less likely in error

Difficult for preceptor to change
diagnosis once made

Learner diagnoses are measured ones,
begins to ↑ with pattern recognition

Figure 5.3 Cognitive Styles of Clinical Reasoning

All aspects of the route from patient history and physical exam through differential diagnosis to treatment, are fertile grounds for discussion with the learner (*see* Figure 5.4). Choose a different one from time to time so that learners can see the scope of considerations involved in the process. Proceed by asking questions: "What if…? Why that test? How sensitive/specific is that test? Will it benefit the patient? What is it likely to be? How do you think the patient will cope with that? What do you think they want?" Agree or disagree, but always share your own thinking process after acknowledging the learner's. Coach the student with questions.

The key is to facilitate the learner developing both their intuition and reasoning. Educationally, the process is one of "integration" or "elaboration" of earlier knowledge being applied to active clinical scenarios. If time does not permit a thorough discussion of the questions raised, deal with them as a case discussion at the end of the day or a small group discussion later on.

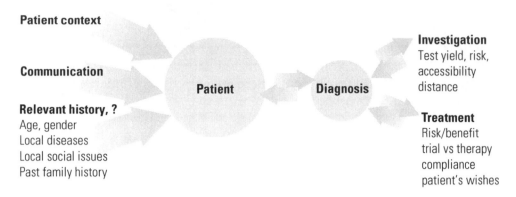

Patient context

Communication

Relevant history, ?
Age, gender
Local diseases
Local social issues
Past family history

Patient

Diagnosis

Investigation
Test yield, risk,
accessibility
distance

Treatment
Risk/benefit
trial vs therapy
compliance
patient's wishes

Figure 5.4 Components of Applied Clinical Reasoning

Supportively question the learner about how they reached their conclusions. Share alternatives, if appropriate. Pass on the need for increased surveillance and urgency with sicker patients. These are all significant learning experiences of things we often do without thinking. Some of these will need to be made explicit, particularly to the novice. The pace at which a given learner will develop appropriate clinical reasoning is highly individualized. We both need to accept the learner's starting point, so that small steps forward can be taken.

As with many educational exercises, an emphasis on patient safety throughout the decision-tree of investigation, treatment and follow-up is a valuable role to model. Facilitating clinical reasoning development occurs daily and requires questioning and reflecting by both parties. Somehow, we all get there in the end and we need to keep an open mind about how the process occurs. It is more like watering a garden than building a shed.

Teaching Small Groups

Teaching small groups in medical education combines both a teaching and facilitating role (*see* Table 5.5). It comes in all forms: discussion groups, tutorials and small group learning. They may be very foreign to many community-based medical educators. The two ends of the educational spectrum are didactic tutorials – "mini lectures" – and the more facilitated, user-friendly small-group discussions. Even a didactic tutorial can be enhanced in ways not possible with larger groups. By using a small-group setting effectively, one can move beyond information sharing to facilitating understanding and knowledge consolidation. Either type of teacher role can still take advantage of one of the key learning attributes of small-group settings. Knowledge is best assimilated by "chewing it over." Students are able to clarify information, to express it in their own terms with their questions. Such information handling leads to better information assimilation: turning information into knowledge.

This process is alternately called "integration" or "elaboration" of knowledge in the educational literature. These terms refer to the students' ability, in a safe learning environment, to take information, discuss it with others, put it into terms they personally understand, relate it to past cases and previous pathophysiology learning. The small-group environment can be used to facilitate this knowledge consolidation even if the main purpose of a didactic tutorial is the transfer of knowledge.

Table 5.5 Components of Small-group Sessions

Basics	
	Who, what do they already know?
	How long is the session?
Preparation	
	Hand-outs, slides
	Learning objectives
Session	
	Introduction
	Be positive
	Discuss objectives
Facilitating	
	Present or have a student present
	Lead discussion
	Encourage quiet members
Summarize/debrief	
	Key learning points
	Things we do not know
	Areas for future learning
	Feedback, plan next one

Tutorial

A common scenario is being asked to teach the students about a given disease. Those are your instructions. There are several practical issues. Who are the learners? What do they already know? How long do you have? Once you have as much information as you will receive, prepare your material, at the appropriate level. Look at your slides and ensure that, for undergraduate learners, some basic physiology and pathology is included, so that it ties into what they have already learned. Prepare hand-outs or electronic documents if information is being shared, so that students can concentrate on the lecture or discussion components rather than constantly taking notes.

Once the session is upon you, begin with introductions if required. Be positive; be enthusiastic about the topic. State why you think it is relevant in your practice and to the learner's education and career. Tell a relevant clinical story on the topic if you have one. Seek relevance from the learners:

> "Have you encountered any diabetic patient yet?"
> "Has anyone had a dislocated shoulder themselves?"
> "Have you had any teaching on this topic yet?"
> "Are there any questions from those sessions which remain confusing?"

Your tone will set up the learning environment. Clarify the topic to be covered, the agreed-upon time of completion and let students know that you want questions raised during the presentation or kept to the end. Seek tacit agreement about proceeding.

Present the material you have prepared. Stop for questions along the way. Involve the learners actively in the topic as best you can. Have some prepared questions of your own to involve learners. Summarize the key points in the last few slides and note areas where further understanding on the topic is necessary. Ask if there are any questions. Consider having several cases to discuss to place the learning in a patient care setting and to involve active participation from the learners. Thank the group for their time. Remember the traditional presentation advice, which is to: "Say what you are going to say, say it and say what you have said."

Small-group Discussions

These sessions are less like a "mini-lecture" and more like a group discussion around a topic and problem-solving as a group. This takes facilitator skills many clinical teachers may not have. The process is similar to the above, but since it involves group members more, it highlights the social milieu and its interactions. Ideal small group size is 6–10 members.

Setting agreed-upon learning objectives/goals is very important. Write them down, so the group can refer back to them as required. As group facilitator, you have more value as a listener than as a speaker. The facilitator does have to "police" the group and limit the overly verbose and draw out the very shy group members. Conflicts and differences may also need to be openly recognized by the facilitator.

The educational benefit of small learning groups is that the learners have a better chance of getting the information into their own terms and knowledge framework. Here, there exists the flexibility to allow learners to relate new information to cases they have seen and to previous knowledge of basic sciences. The learners are able to chew the topic around and become familiar with it, unlike in a lecture where they must swallow it whole or fall behind, sometimes with little assimilation. How do we facilitate such learning?

The most important task is setting up a comfortable interactive learning environment. We do this by not beginning like a lecture, but we do need to set clear learning objectives. We should also lay out the expectation that this is not a lecture and everyone is welcome to participate. Certainly, if there will be marks assigned to this for participation, the students need to know this.

Our role is to set up the topic of interest and encourage discussion by asking about related clinical cases and learning issues related to them. The facilitator can raise these issues and listen. Ensure that someone does not dominate the discussion and ensure the quiet group member is not left out. The key to developing an interactive group is to set up a supportive learning environment. The facilitator does not dominate the discussion; when one does that, it is an admission that they are willing to do all the talking and the work of the session. Others will sit back and relax if there is nothing for them to do. Resist this type of "leadership." A good facilitator needs group leadership skills, but portrays them with more questioning, encouragement and listening and less speaking. This may be a challenge for a "take-charge" personality.

During the course of the discussion, you might make lists of problem areas that need further exploration if this is to be a series of tutorials. The written list, despite coming from the small group members themselves, is a composite of all their learning needs and confers a degree of anonymity and learner-safety. It also gives a clear visual pathway proceeding toward the learning objectives. Role-playing may also assist in active participation. Move the roles around the room. Let participants reflect and comment on their performance if they wish.

Upon completion of the session, thank the group for their participation. Ask what went well, were the objectives met and what could we do better next time? Use these suggestions to plan the next session.

SUMMARY

Teaching can be a gratifying addition to a career in community-based medicine. It shares many of the same qualities as patient care: patience, humor, challenges and relationship. It helps us keep up to date and participate in the development of the next generation of physicians. Students are a part of the larger community to which we contribute. Discomfort in some areas of teaching is not uncommon and can be addressed by seeking out meaningful faculty development. It is a bit like seeing children you have delivered grow up in your community. The students eventually become your colleagues and there is a lifelong relationship in the background. Ultimately, we want to pass on to our learners the example and skills to think critically and listen well.

FURTHER READING

Colliver J. Educational theory and medical education practice: a cautionary note for medical school faculty. *Acad Med.* 2002; **77**(12): 1217-20.

DaRosa D, Skeff K, Frienland J, *et al.* Barriers to effective teaching. *Acad Med.* 2011; **86**(4): 1-7.

Dent J. AMEE Guide no 26: clinical teaching in ambulatory care settings: making the most of learning opportunities with outpatients. *Med Teach.* 2005; **27**(4): 302-15.

Haglund M, Rot M, Cooper N, *et al.* Resilience in the third year of medical school: a prospective study of associations between stressful events occurring during clinical rotations and student well-being. *Acad Med.* 2009; **84**(2): 258-68.

Harden R, Crosby J. AMEE guide no 20: the good teacher is more than a lecturer - the twelve roles of the teacher. *Med Teach.* 2000; **22**(4): 334-47.

Hatem C, Searle N, Gunderman R, *et al.* The educational attributes and responsibilities of effective medical educators. *Acad Med.* 2011; **86**(4): 1-7.

Hoff T, Pohl H, Bartfield J. Creating a learning environment to produce competent residents: the roles of culture and context. *Acad Med.* 2004; **79**(6): 532-9.

Leung G, Johnston J, Evidence-based medical education - quo vadis? *J Eval Clin Pract.* 2006; **12**(3): 353-64.

MacAllister L, Higgs J, Smith D. Facing and managing dilemmas as a clinical educator. *High Ed Research Dev.* 2008; **27**(1): 1-13.

May W, Park J, Lee J. A ten-year review of the literature on the use of standardized patients. *Med Teach.* 2009; **31**: 487-92.

McLeod P, Harden R. Clinical teaching strategies for physicians. *Med Teach.* 1985; **7**(2): 173-89.

Osmun W, Copeland J. The occasional teacher. Part 1: teaching in a rural setting. *Can J Rural Med.* 2010; **15**(4): 162-3.

Perkoff G. Teaching medicine in the ambulatory setting: an idea whose time may have finally come. *New Engl J Med.* 1986; **314**(1): 27-31.

Ramani S. Twelve tips to promote excellence in medical teaching. *Med Teach.* 2006; **28**(1): 19-23.

Ramani S, Leinster S. AMEE guide no 43: teaching in the clinical environment. *Med Teach.* 2008; **30**: 347-64.

Schultz KW, Kirby J, Delva D, *et al.* Medical students' and residents' preferred site characteristics and preceptor behaviours for learning in the ambulatory setting: a cross-sectional survey. *BMC Med Educ.* 2004; **4**: 12.

Seehusen D, Miser W. Teaching the outstanding medical learner. *Fam Med.* 2006; **37**(10): 731-5.

Walters L, Greenhill J, Ash J, *et al.* Longitudinal Integrated Clinical Placements; time for a theoretical framework. 2011, in press.

Whitcomb M. More on competency-based education. *Acad Med.* 2004; **79**(6): 493-4.

Time Management

Cape J. Consultation length, patient-estimated consultation length and satisfaction with the consultation. *Br J Gen Pract.* 2002; **52**: 1004-6.

Dugdale D, Epstein R, Pantilat S. Time and patient-physician relationship. *JGIM.* 1999; **14**: S34-40.

Mauksch L, Dugdale D, Dodson S, *et al.* Relationship, communication and efficiency in the medical encounter: creating a clinical model from a literature review. *Arch Intern Med.* 2008; **168**(13): 1387–95.

Wilson A, Childs S. Effect of interventions aimed at changing the length of primary care physicians' consultation. *Cochrane Database Syst Rev.* 2009.

Small-Group Teaching

Jones V, Holland A, Oldmeadow W. Inductive teaching method – an alternative method for small group learning. *Med Teach.* 2008; **30**: e246–9.

Kilroy D. Problem-based learning. *Emerg Med J.* 2004; **21**: 422–3.

Kolars J, Gruppen L, Traber P, *et al.* The effect of student and teacher centered small group learning in medical school on knowledge acquisition, retention and application. *Med Teach.* 1997; **19**(1): 53–7.

Lewin L, Lanken P. Longitudinal small-group learning during the first clinical year. *Fam Med.* 2004; **36**: S3–8.

Lochner L, Gijselaers W. Improving lecture skills: a time-efficient 10 step pedagogical consultation method for medical teachers in healthcare professions. *Med Teach.* 2011; **33**: 131–6.

Nasmith L, Daigle N. Small-group teaching in patient education. *Med Teach.* 1996; **18**(3): 209–11.

O'Neil P, Willis S, Jones A. A model of how students link problem-based learning with clinical experience through "elaboration." *Acad Med.* 2002; **77**(6): 552–61.

Rotem A, Manzie P. How to use small groups in medical education. *Med Teach.* 1980; **2**: 80–7.

Steniert Y. Twelve tips for effective small-group teaching in the health professions. *Med Teach.* 1996; **18**(3): 203–7.

Communication Skills

Aspegren K. MEME Guide no 1: teaching and learning communication skills in medicine – a review with quality grading of articles. *Med Teach.* 1999; **21**(6): 563–70.

Gordon G. Defining the skills underlying communication competence. *Semin Med Pract.* 2002; **5**(3): 21–8.

Laidlaw A, Hart J. Communication skills: an essential component of medical curricula. Part 1: assessment of clinical communication: AMEE guide no 51. *Med Teach.* 2011; **33**: 6–8.

Macguire P, Pitceathly C. Key communication skills and how to acquire them. *BMJ.* 2002; **325**: 697–700.

Perron N, Sommer J, Hudelson P, *et al.* Clinical supervisors' perceived needs for teaching communication skill in clinical practice. *Med Teach.* 2009; **31**: e316–22.

Roensberg E, Lussier M, Beaudoin C. Lessons for clinicians from physician–patient communication literature. *Arch Fam Med.* 1997; **6**: 279–83.

Smith R. *The Patient's Story: an evidence based method.* 2nd ed. Philadelphia: Lippincott Williams & Wilkins; 2001.

Stewart M, Brown J, Weston W, *et al. Patient Centered Medicine: transforming the clinical method.* Thousand Oaks, California; Sage Publications: 1995.

Tamblyn R, Abrahamowicz M, Dauphinee D, *et al.* Physician scores on a national clinical skills examination as predictors of complaints to medical regulatory authorities. *JAMA.* 2007; **298**(9): 993–1001.

Van dalen J, Van Hout J, Wolfhagen H, *et al.* Factors influencing the effectiveness of communication skills training: programme contents outweigh teachers' skills. *Med Teach.* 1999; **21**(3): 308–10.

Clinical Reasoning

Carraccio C, Bradley J, Nixon J, *et al.* From the education bench to the clinical bedside: translating the Dreyfus developmental model to the learning of clinical skills. *Acad Med.* 2008; **83**(8): 761–7.

Dequeker J, Jaspaert R. Teaching problem-solving and clinical reasoning: 20 years' experience with video-supported small-group learning. *Med Educ.* 1998; **32**: 384–9.

Kassirer J. Teaching clinical reasoning: case-based and coached. *Acad Med.* 2010; **85**(7): 1118–24.

Kilroy D. Problem-based learning. *Emerg Med J.* 2004; **21**: 411–13.

O'Neil P, Wills S, Jones A. A model of how students link problem-based learning with clinical experience through "elaboration." *Acad Med.* 2002; **77**(6): 552–61.

Radomski N, Russell J. Integrated case learning: teaching clinical reasoning. *Adv Health Sci Educ Theory Pract.* 2010; **15**(2): 251–64.

Windish D. Teaching medical students clinical reasoning skills. *Acad Med.* 2000; **75**(1): 90.

6

Bedside Teaching

Michael Betts and David Rosenthal

Bedside clinical teaching is returning to consideration as a teaching tool in medical education. During the past 30 years, its use has declined, overshadowed by an explosion in both theoretical knowledge and technology. Notwithstanding those changes, new knowledge and technology need to be applied appropriately and economically to the management of live patients.

Bedside teachers function in a special environment. While some people involved in healthcare speak of "clients," experienced physicians speak of patients. This is, in part, because they understand that when ill, people usually behave "patiently." They often do not have the capacity to behave otherwise. They carry a unique level of trust in their doctors which, along with their illness, places them in the hands of their physician for their well-being. Doctors in training must understand these dynamics at the bedside and learn, not only about the symptoms, signs and management of disease, but also the patient's reaction to them. They also need to understand and apply principles of safety and quality in healthcare to develop an understanding of patient-centered care.

AD HOC vs SCHEDULED ROUNDS

All experienced clinicians take short-cuts and tailor their clinical exam to the needs at hand. That is a very different starting point than for most novice learners, who cannot distinguish the "always done" from the "sometimes needed" parts of a clinical scenario. If we are carrying out our regular clinical work and come across an interesting finding, we should share it – bringing a student in to listen to respiratory crackles can be invaluable. We should do this as often as we can, even though some learners have not yet mastered normal findings and they may not appreciate completely unusual ones.

We play a different role if our role that day is to teach a systematic approach to a part of the physical exam: inspect, auscultate, percuss, etc. This is a time for the preceptor to step back and even consult the clinical exam text used by the learners. That way we can give a broad-based approach to the exam, from which the learner can subsequently adopt their own malleable "short forms." A systematic approach to the physical exam is quite different from sharing positive findings in our day-to-day clinical teaching, but both are invaluable bedside teaching components.

Scheduled Clinical Teaching Rounds

The timing of the bedside teaching session depends largely on patient and environmental circumstances. Sensible consideration of hospital routines, the patient journey, and the patient's visitor program should enable proper timing. Prior to entering the patient's room, a brief but measured description of the patient and their circumstances should be given to learners. In particular, it is important to outline any areas of potential sensitivity in the patient's presentation, personality, or in the impending physical examination. Instructors should always model advocacy regarding patient dignity and comfort. Learners also receive advice regarding the tasks to be assigned, together with a cross-check on their previous clinical exposure.

The outcomes from a bedside clinical teaching session will vary, depending on the learners' academic level and this will impact on planning the session. Therefore, some reference is necessary to the learners' curriculum and to an understanding of the norms expected from learners at that point in time. This may influence planning: for example, junior students may essentially receive demonstration and supervision of particular techniques in a small well-defined area, while more senior learners may have a task that is both wider and deeper.

There is no correct number of patients to encounter. The mix of clinical teaching/disease teaching should not be set in stone. The curiosity of myasthenia gravis should not necessarily occupy the same teaching time as might diabetes mellitus, interesting though the myasthenia could be. The mix is determined by the disease, and to some extent, on the emphasis placed on it within the learners' curriculum – another reason for teaching clinicians allowing themselves time to be familiar with the curriculum.

Patient Involvement

Most patients will allow teaching to occur in their presence following a courteous request and an explanation of the role from the teaching doctor. This should be tempered with a consideration of the patient's symptoms such as pain or nausea, apprehension or disillusionment. The process of requesting patient involvement by the preceptor occurs privately before any teaching session and should not be hurried, and a negative answer should be accepted with grace. It is best to allow some time for the patient to process a request for involvement, as well as some discussion, in order to successfully understand their role.

The aim of a teaching physician is to use a bedside encounter with a patient to gain a positive learning outcome for learners. A sound personal relationship between teaching doctor and patient assists the process. When agreement to proceed has been secured, the essentials of the patient's situation can be discussed with them, together with an outline of the tasks which the learner(s) will be expected to undertake. We should not forget that, in rural areas, patients hope that their contribution to teaching will result in more learners returning to their area as practising doctors. The patients are given the option to terminate any student exam when they wish. They are asked to let the preceptor know how the student treated them and are encouraged to be a part of the feedback loop – given confidentially to the preceptor after the session with the learner is completed. "Was the student respectful and gentle, or otherwise?"

Involving the patient in the teaching process, rather than as someone on whom to demonstrate techniques etc. is a matter of judgment. An intelligent, pain-free and insightful patient may well be a useful adjunct to the learning session; a less understanding patient may be a hindrance. However, if the teacher can intervene where necessary, this in itself is instructive. Where the lesson involves history-taking, clearly the patient must be involved in both telling the story and indicating where symptoms lie. Teachers should draw attention to the human mystery of variability in presentation of disease.

HOW TO PROCEED

Historically, the introducing physician enters the room ahead of anyone else. This is important because the patient looks to the treating physician to have influence over all that is happening to them, including teaching. A courteous greeting, followed by introductions is a necessity. If a particular examination technique is to be taught, it is appropriate for the teacher to demonstrate it, and with the patient's consent, to have learners follow the example given. However, many learners are transitioning to clinical practice and a bedside teaching session can be useful in enabling a learner to combine basic history and examination with a demonstration of clinical reasoning. That will generally result in other learners in the group observing and drawing their own conclusions regarding the exercise.

This process can take time and it is useful for teachers to plan the best use of patients' commitment during a bedside teaching session. It is helpful to outline the aims of the session to learners and to refer back to them if necessary, especially when approaching different patients. Some questions from students may warrant out-of-session discussion, in order to maximize clinical outcomes and use of patient commitment. It is always a challenge to maintain interest for the members of the group who are not actively involved in a clinical task. They can be given questions about a particular case, e.g. explaining pathophysiology, or overall disease management, or a contemplation of the impact of hospitalization on the patient – and contribute to discussion from a considered perspective.

Where there is only one learner it does not matter who goes first as more than one examination can occur, particularly with exercises such as auscultation, joint or skin examination, and they can be repeated as needed. With a larger class, we suggest that the teacher specify the task and that the task should be small and specific. For example "inspect the abdomen" or "measure the visual acuity" breaks down the exam's component parts so that less time is spent in non-activity by the other learners. If the first learner finds a positive finding, those following can be instructed on what to see or hear.

DEBRIEFING

It is useful to track the learner's level of interest and engagement and, if problems are present, to be innovative in managing them. "Time out" in sessions or an adjournment to sit and discuss the cases and questions may be useful. As a matter of principle, we suggest that feedback is best given when the case is fresh in the learner's mind. Anything which is not understood from the case should be the backbone of debriefing, as correct information gleaned from the teaching case is the basis for on-going learning. The debriefing is essentially a measure of what has been understood and where that experience fits in the learner's current state of knowledge.

At any teaching event, learners are keen to understand how clinicians "join the dots." Inevitably, that means teachers have an opportunity to describe, not only what they do, but also how they think in particular situations. A typical example of this is the intellectual approach to the neurological case in which a differential diagnosis of the lesion is made, together with an assessment of its neurological level. Experienced teachers have much to contribute to these discussions. Anecdotal teaching and "story telling" have, along with bedside teaching, recently been somewhat out of fashion. We believe that graphic clinical experiences, whether they are positive or negative, whether they are personal or second-hand, are nodal points in the life of a clinician. Rarely are they not instructive and, used judiciously, they are valuable teaching instruments.

Suggestions for clinical teachers include taking short notes for use in the student debriefing afterwards. As this is done, take note of learners' styles and difficulties and try to develop suggestions for later use. This can be difficult, but practice makes the task easier. In addition, some conceptual understanding of how people learn and how it is hoped that learning occurs within the teacher's institution is most useful. It is useful to practice techniques that ensure the session does not become bogged in minutiae. Finally, difficult questions will inevitably arise. If an answer cannot immediately be provided, a follow-up approach will be needed.

SUMMARY

Bedside clinical teaching remains a useful way of contextualizing the teaching of medicine using real patients. Probably, the difference between its uses now, compared with years ago, is that, currently, teaching clinicians may be more familiar with medical education and the facilitation of small groups. As well, the assessment of clinical signs and symptoms stands dwarfed in the modern forest of CT scans and MRI angiograms. But it is in bedside teaching where we encounter the sick patient. Listening to their story and sharing a clinical exam is at the core of the patient–doctor relationship and trust. It all comes down to the patient, and bedside teaching reminds us of that imperative. Learners also need to master the clinical exam holistically, while negotiating respect with the patient, as neither of these will be out of date anytime soon.

FURTHER READING

Janick R, Fletcher K. Teaching at the bedside: a new model. *Med Teach.* 2002; **25**(2): 127–30.

Nair B, Coughlan J, Hensley M. Student and patient perspectives on bedside teaching. *Med Educ.* 1997; **31**: 341–6.

7

The Learner's Perspective

David VanderBurgh and Aaron Orkin

PROFESSORS, PARENTS AND PARTNERS: A NOVEL TYPOLOGY OF COMMUNITY PRECEPTORS

Starting a new rotation is daunting. It keeps us up at night, we just do not like it, and as far as we know, most other residents and medical students do not care for it much either. Attempting to impress a palliative care specialist on a Sunday, and an orthopedic surgeon on a Monday, brings uncertainty and stress. As family medicine residents, we bumped from one rotation to another every month or two, and the beginning of each rotation felt like starting a new job. Stress lay in unknown expectations and uncertainty, not only about our clinical knowledge but also about the variable behaviors and expectations of our preceptors.

Leaving the teaching hospital to start a small-town family medicine rotation felt a bit like coming home. We developed a familiarity with these community preceptors, their expectations and their behaviors, and spent enough time in these settings to understand the culture of our preceptors. We observed them and found patterns. This is not to suggest that community-based preceptors are a uniform bunch, but they do display a certain range of behaviors with learners. Over time, we have refined our approach to the community-based preceptor to arrive at a categorization or typology of community preceptors and their behaviors.

The purpose of this chapter is to share this typology, not only with preceptors and medical educators, but also with medical learners. We introduce and describe the three broad types of community preceptor: the professor, the parent, and the partner. We explore their strengths, weaknesses and varieties.

We hope our approach to the varieties of community preceptors might permit learners to recognize their own preceptor's behaviors, identify them as representative of one of these types, and understand how they can gain the most from the rotation. This chapter might also assist preceptors seeking to be more mindful in their teaching, or those interested in exploring different teaching styles.

The box vignettes presented with each section capture representative experiences with each type of preceptor. For each preceptor, we provide a vignette to explore one potential strength and weakness. We have tried to outline what certain types of preceptors might say in a particular situation, but in our box vignettes – as in real educational interactions – the tone is paramount. How things are said might be as important as what things are said. The vignettes all deal with the same clinical scenario: the presentation and management of an uncomplicated anterior shoulder dislocation.

Throughout the text, the words "he" and "she" are used interchangeably and without gender bias to refer to preceptors and students. All behavioral typologies have been observed in both male and female preceptors.

THE PROFESSOR

The professor's key attribute is that he believes there to be a correct answer to every medical question. He is directive in his approach, and may outline for the learner, not only his rotation objectives, but also clear ideas of what a physician should be. As a learner, a fairly effective approach to determining whether a preceptor fits the professorial mold is to observe that the more medical adages and eponyms used by the preceptor, the more likely he is a professorial preceptor.

For some learners, a directive, professorial style is comforting and motivating. Transition from the textbooks and into the clinic can be challenging for some trainees. Application processes at most medical schools place an overwhelming emphasis on book-learning abilities and many medical learners have limited experience in demonstrating their intellectual capacities outside the walls of a conventional classroom. A professor-preceptor returns the medical learner to a place of comfort, and likely to a place of strength. With a professor-preceptor, there exists a correct answer, and if a learner reads, studies, works and tries enough, he will find, remember and regurgitate this correct answer. The learner will also rejoice from the positive feedback of a correct response – we certainly did. The professorial preceptor, as shown in Box 7.1, can provide learners with a useful approach to a clinical problem without having the learner look it up themselves. These titbits of knowledge, approaches to problems, and memory aids need to be handed down through preceptors and presentations, because formal reading around a clinical problem seldom yields these useful tricks.

Professor-preceptors also tend to place expectations of expertise and proficiency on themselves and their colleagues. What the professor-preceptor knows, she knows well, and a learner who find himself with such a supervisor can learn tremendous amounts by permitting the preceptor to teach about the medical concepts and approaches she knows best. Professorial preceptors also

---

BOX 7.1 The Anterior Shoulder Dislocation

Trainee: I think that this patient has an anterior shoulder dislocation.

Professor-preceptor: Okay, good. There are three risks I always consider before doing a reduction. From distal to proximal: there are risks to the limb, to the joint and to the person. Can you name them?

Trainee: Ummm, how about for the limb there's neurovascular compromise, for the joint there's the risk of a fracture, and with the person ...umm.

Professor-preceptor: Consider the sedation also...

Trainee: Oh! Airway compromise, allergic reaction...I'll remember that approach!

Professor-preceptor: See, the clinical problem is about the whole patient and everything that goes with the problem – sedation risks are part of the problem and need to be considered from the beginning.

---

tend to demonstrate a willingness to provide feedback and demand excellence and rigor from a learner at any level. Learners who feel their professional or clinical growth may have reached a plateau, are looking for a new challenge or who want someone to provide criticism tend to do well with an engaged preceptor of this type. These preceptors also tend to be useful contacts to help with rounds, presentations, research undertakings or other academic responsibilities.

The professor-preceptor can be appropriate and tame in her approach. However, the "being right" behavior can spin out of control in two main ways. First, a preceptor may extend her area of expertise beyond the medical world to all spheres of life. The preceptor may share with her learner the right way to raise her children, the right stocks to invest in, and the right type of yoghurt to buy (seriously, this actually happened)! We imagine this type of "expertise creep" can emerge in other types of preceptors, but from our experience, it has been most pronounced in educators who adopt a professorial approach. For some learners, these behaviors can be perceived as charming eccentricity. For others, it can be jarring and produce a sense of inadequacy and stress. Do I have to be like my preceptor if I am going to be a good family doctor?

Second, in this role, preceptors can risk developing an adversarial relationship with their learner. It is within the broad category of professor-preceptors that the timeless and excruciating practice of "pimping," or adversarial quizzing, emerged in medical education. In his 1989 JAMA piece, "The Art of Pimping," Brancati pokes fun at both preceptors and learners by outlining the rules of engagement and strategies for "pimping." From the preceptor's side, questions may fall into one of five categories: 1. arcane points of history; 2. teleology and metaphysics; 3. exceedingly broad questions; 4. eponyms; or, 5. technical points of laboratory research. The experienced and astute learner, Brancati quips, has two possible defenses for the challenging question: the dodge or the bluff. The vignette in Box 7.2 exposes how a professorial preceptor can find sport in quizzing their learner, and the tension that can result. By holding the right answers, a professorial preceptor runs risk of fostering an adversarial relationship with their learner and a competitive, not co-operative, work environment.

BOX 7.2 The Anterior Shoulder Dislocation

Trainee: I think that reduction went really well. Wow!

Professor-preceptor: Okay. There are at least six methods to reduce a shoulder described by Kelly in the *Canadian Journal of Rural Medicine*. What are they?

Trainee: We just did the one we where you apply traction and move the arm so that it is in a throwing position, like if the patient was about to throw a ball or scratch his head. Umm…

Professor-preceptor: Yes. But what's it called? Someone at your level should know this! The Milch technique. Who was Milch?

THE PARENT

Of the three types of preceptor we outline here, parent-preceptors are by far the most likely to ask their learner over for dinner. The parent-preceptor is a caregiver and supporter. Oftentimes, this type of preceptor shows extensive interest in your life outside medicine, asking about your upbringing, your family, your spouse, your pets and your hobbies. A parent-preceptor will be interested in your work life balance, your coping strategies for the stresses of medical education and practice. He will be interested in getting you access to both the yoga studio or shinny league in town. As an educator, the parent-preceptor is supportive, and may – like a real parent – be more lenient or overbearing than he ought to be.

For many learners, a parent-type preceptor develops an environment conducive to inquiry and academic risk-taking. A learner feels supported, safe and comfortable to ask questions they may be embarrassed to ask elsewhere. Consider the example of the anterior shoulder dislocation in Box 7.3. The astute parent-preceptor notices not only the patient's needs but also that his student is struggling with the case, not for academic reasons but for personal ones. Finding a preceptor who can help guide the learner through processes like this is an important part of the student's success and transition into self-reflective independent practice.

BOX 7.3 The Anterior Shoulder Dislocation

Trainee: I think that this patient has an anterior shoulder dislocation.

Parent-preceptor: Okay, good diagnosis. But you look pale…are you okay?

Trainee: Umm, yeah, I think his shoulder needs to be reduced.

Parent-preceptor: Good, but just hold on for a second. What's wrong?

Trainee: It is just that my shoulder got dislocated skiing when I was a kid and it was awful. Every time I see a patient with dislocated shoulder I feel like I'm going to pass out.

Parent-preceptor: Okay, let's take some time to talk about that after we do this reduction. Would that be alright?

Trainee: Okay.

Trusting relationships built between parent-preceptors and learners can be a very important part of medical education as learners seek to find experienced mentors and supervisors with whom they can speak more candidly and honestly about their fears and choices. The learner may feel safe to discuss negative experiences they have had elsewhere in their medical training. Debriefing critical events, medical errors, or challenging learning experiences can be a formative piece of medical education and the parent-preceptor often creates an environment to discuss these previous experiences. Parent-preceptors want to see their trainees succeed and find professional and personal fulfilment, and are often able to provide useful and trusted advice about career choices, choosing a residency program, or exploring locum opportunities.

Still, the parent-preceptor may be overbearing. "Helicopter parent" is a pop-culture term for a hovering mom and dad, who remain too close, never out of reach. Parent-preceptors can become helicopter preceptors who hover over their trainees, waiting to pluck them out of a difficult spot, smoothing their learning-experiences and shielding them from "difficult" patients, cumbersome paperwork, or overly onerous call duties (*see* Box 7.4). While we believe

---

BOX 7.4 The Anterior Shoulder Dislocation

Trainee: I think this patient has an anterior shoulder dislocation.

Parent-preceptor: Oh, is that Mr. Smith?

Trainee: Yeah, how did you know?

Parent-preceptor: Oh, he comes in all the time! He dislocates his shoulder intentionally and presents to the emergency department. He can reduce it easily himself. Narcotic addiction is the main problem. Don't worry about this, I will go see him.

Trainee: Are you sure?

Parent-preceptor: Yeah, I'll handle it.

---

that this protectionism is exercised with the best of intentions, it can have an adverse effect on the learner. Just as a sheltered teen will struggle significantly to adjust when they leave home for the first time, an insulated learner will also struggle as an independent practitioner. "Difficult" patients encountered by the learner almost invariably represent important educational opportunities.

THE PARTNER

In the role of partner, the staff physician exhibits the behaviors of a co-ordinator or guide for their learner. Conventional medical education hierarchies might dissolve as the learner is treated as a partner in learning and patient care and the learner become an intellectual equal and colleague. Questions are often reflected back to the trainee, as the preceptor urges the trainee to wrestle with the same clinical questions faced by the community-based physician. There are no easy answers.

There are pros and cons to this type of educator. Returning to our vignette, the anterior shoulder dislocation, the preceptor responds to the learner's question by reflecting it back to the learner. This approach can initiate a meaningful discussion between learner and preceptor about an area of controversy or practice variability. In a case like this, particularly effective preceptors of this type will succeed in having the learner arrive at an appropriate choice, not by providing an answer, but by providing the learner with enough confidence to make a decision herself. Generally, partner-preceptors make learners feel empowered and important (*see* Box 7.5). Learners may feel trusted and their ability to reason through clinical problems is respected. Caring for patients can feel like a real and rewarding collaboration between the learner and her preceptor.

BOX 7.5 The Anterior Shoulder Dislocation

Trainee: I think that this patient has an anterior shoulder dislocation.

Partner-preceptor: Okay. What's your plan?

Trainee: I think his shoulder needs to be reduced and I'm ready to do it with you. I've encountered some debate about whether pre-reduction X-ray films are necessary. What is your practice?

Partner-preceptor: Good question. What is your practice when it comes to pre-reduction films?

Preceptors who succeed in this role can enhance learning experiences by partnering in educational initiatives as well as patient care. For example, while debriefing at the end of a clinic, a partner-type educator might share educational responsibilities by saying something like, "Okay, there were four key questions that came up today. How about you look up two, and I'll look up two, and we'll chat about them tomorrow."

Some sources suggest that learners respond positively to this type of educator. In 2004, Shultz published one of the largest surveys of medical student and resident experiences, questioning over 3000 Ontario learners regarding what site characteristics and preceptor behaviors most enhanced their learning in an ambulatory setting. What was the number-one factor positively affecting learner experience? A preceptor who was open to questions from his student or resident. Parent-preceptors and professor-preceptors can also be open to questions from their learner, but a preceptor who positions himself in partnership with his student not only creates a safe environment for questions but also allows learners to expand on their confidence and attempt to answer questions as well. The partner-preceptor also creates the greatest opportunities for her learner to do the teaching, meaning that partner-preceptors might find their teaching experiences reciprocated and rewarding.

Still, the partner is not the ideal educator for all learners or all contexts, and attempts to adopt partnering behaviors can lead astray. With this mode of education, the student is often expected to be self-directed and confident, and there may be unclear expectations from the learner's perspective. Some thrive under this freedom and independence. Other learners can flounder, however, and need clearer objectives or expectations to be set out. The partner-preceptor might sometimes serve these trainees well by taking cues from other types of preceptor. Further, for some learners, a partnership with their staff can lead to a lack of confidence in their supervisor. And, as we see in Shultz and others' work, medical trainees rank having a preceptor whom they believe to have a high command of their specialty as very important. For some learners, especially early in training, a preceptor who knows, offers a right answer and is purposive and directive in their approach can inspire confidence.

Just because the preceptor–student relationship has become an effective partnership does not mean that the preceptor's primary concerns or interests should be allowed to guide the educational process. Overly collegial partner-preceptors can erode the quality of learning by shifting the educational focus of the partnership attention away from the learner's primary concerns. In treating the interaction as a genuinely collegial partnership, the preceptor's preoccupations can become too important. The preceptor's interest in billing codes or practice management, for example, may not be appropriate for learners in earlier stages of their training (*see* Box 7.6).

BOX 7.6 The Anterior Shoulder Dislocation

Trainee: Wow. That reduction went really well.

Partner-preceptor: Yeah, I really like it. And you can bill for the assessment, the intra-articular injection, the reduction, and the procedural sedation.

SUMMARY

Each of the preceptor types presented in this chapter plays an important and formative role in a community-based family practice setting. None of these types is more "good;" none is more "bad." Together with their colleagues and patients, this typology of preceptors and their learners might be seen as a delicate, balanced ecosystem. Its efficacy depends upon the diversity of people and their behaviors. Ultimately, good training relies on finding and interacting with all kinds of preceptors. It is our experience that a special, educationally formative and positive rotation does not emerge from any single factor or any universally reproducible preceptor behavior. There is no one way to be a great preceptor and each learner will respond differently to different approaches.

The repetition of the same clinical scenario in the box vignettes throughout this chapter demonstrate how the same clinical moment can produce profoundly different educational and experiential outcomes with different preceptors, and emphasizes how many ways we can get it right or get it wrong. A truly exceptional preceptor, perhaps, can learn to transition between different behavioral types to draw the strengths of each type of preceptoring while finding ways to avoid the pitfalls of each. More realistically, good preceptors are aware of the weaknesses of their teaching behaviors and teach to their own strengths.

A final piece of this transition is also the realization that the end of our time as designated medical learners does not mark the end of our time as learners in a medical environment. The typology we have developed represents an attempt to manage our perplexity in the face of new rotations and preceptor behaviors. We believe that, as we transition from trainees to independent physicians, our new perspective may lead to the development, discovery and description of new approaches and preceptor types, hybrids and mosaicisims. And, as staff, we will explore whether preceptors are equally perplexed by their trainees. As preceptors, will we still lie awake at night before a new educational block, anxious about the new learner joining us in the morning?

FURTHER READING

Brancati F. The art of pimping. *JAMA*. 1989; **262**(1): 88–9.

Epstein RM, Cole DR, Gawinski BA, *et al*. How students learn from community-based preceptors. *Arch Fam Med*. 1998; **7**(2): 149–54.

Goertzen J, Stewart M, Weston W, *et al*. Effective teaching behaviours of rural family medicine preceptors. *CMAJ*. 1995; **153**(2): 161–8.

Kelly, L. The occasional shoulder reduction. *Can J Rural Med*. 2007; **12**(2): 103–10.

Latessa R, Beaty N, Colvin G, *et al*. Family medicine community preceptors: different from other physician specialties? *Fam Med*. 2008; **40**(2): 96–101.

Leone-Perkins M, Schnuth RL, Lipsky MS. Students' evaluations of teaching and learning experiences at community- and residency-based practices. *Fam Med*. 1999; **31**(8): 572–7.

Mash B, de Villiers M. Community-based training in family medicine – a different paradigm. *Med Educ*. 1999; **33**(10): 725–9.

Paukert J. How medical students and residents describe the roles and characteristics of their influential teachers. *Acad Med*. 2000; **75**(8): 843–5.

Schultz KW, Kirby J, Delva D, *et al*. Medical students' and residents' preferred site characteristics and preceptor behaviours for learning in the ambulatory setting: a cross-sectional survey. *BMC Med Educ*. 2004; **4**: 12.

8

The Difficult Learner

Len Kelly

Most learners we teach do just fine and enhance our day-to-day practice. Encountering a difficult learner can have a temporary or long-term effect on our enjoyment and willingness to teach. A problem learner can range from a student who needs more teaching and supervision, but who eventually makes good progress, to a resident who has more deep-seated issues or who just does not fit into your practice. In this latter scenario, the educational agenda has become derailed and, try as we might, we cannot get it back on track and we will need strategies for developing an educational diagnosis. We will need help to clarify an effective educational strategy. Encountering such frustrations is rare, but they will be draining. The time we set aside for our clinical supervision role will expand dramatically when working with a learner in difficulty. Since patient care itself can be draining, the last thing we feel we need is another "chore." Having a systematic approach will help. We will look at dealing with the difficult learner with this in mind.

There are times that the problem arises from the program which has poorly administered the rotation and the learner arrives frustrated and, not at their best, at an unexpected time or incorrect address. Alternatively, the preceptor may be the source of the "teaching difficulty." If the preceptor is encountering professional or personal stress, they may be overly negative, critical or impatient and not up to the task of supervising a learner. Clearly, these issues cannot be placed at the learner's door, but they will certainly negatively affect the learning experience. These later scenarios seem self-evident and even a break from teaching responsibilities may be in order. For the purposes of this discussion, we shall acknowledge that such preceptor- and program-based issues create learning problems which need to be identified and addressed, but will focus on learner-based learning difficulties. These are the most confounding for the community-based preceptor, who often will falsely initially feel their teaching is at fault. The good will and teaching confidence of the preceptor can quickly drain away when faced with learner-based difficulties.

INCIDENCE

How common are difficult learners? The literature estimate is generally based on self-reporting by program directors and lies at 5–15%. One US military 3-year family medicine program did a review of 25 years of their residents and found a 9% incidence of "residents in trouble." This 2006 study by Reamy noted that, with remediation and counseling, the majority of these residents were able to graduate. Interestingly, while knowledge deficits accounted for 27%, the majority of problems fell into attitudinal categories (interpersonal conflicts, substance abuse and psychiatric illness). In their review, they found that summative evaluations rarely identified any of these 21 residents in trouble! The issues were identified through program directors dealing with complaints and behavior reports. Clearly, community-based medical educators' mid-term and summative evaluations are an important opportunity for identification of learners in need of help.

A British study in 2002 by Sayer *et al* looked at medical students who had failed rotations and noted a wide variation in causes, but a cluster of subjects found difficulty around communication skills. A 1999 survey of 300 internal medicine residency program directors in the US described their estimated rate of problem residents at 7%. These program directors reinforced that problem residents do not self-identify. They are typically identified through direct observation in clinical settings by the chief resident or attending physician. As in Reamy's 25-year retrospective study, these program administrators identified that poorly completed clinical summative evaluations hampered their ability to convince the resident that their behavior was problematic.

Learners experience depression and anxiety disorders three times more often than the general population, according to Earle's study. Her 2005 study of Ontario family medicine residents found that 8% of them required a leave of absence for mental health issues. Private or deep-seated issues will need referral, and typically that will mean to a physician or mental health worker not involved in the teaching program. It is important to ensure that the learner has access to time off to access whatever support they need. Medical educational is like clinical medicine in that safety comes first, for the patient, learner and the preceptor. All educational programs have access to mental health services and we need to be sure the learner knows they can be accessed confidentially.

These studies hold two important messages for community-based medical educators. The first is the realization that they are in the best position to identify problem learners, as they see them in clinical settings where problems surface. The second is the importance that mid-term and summative evaluations can play for the learner in difficulty. We must be aware of and document behaviors, and contact program personnel early in this process.

CONCEPTUAL FRAMEWORK

Of the several theoretical frameworks in the literature, the simplest and most intuitive has been developed by Steinert, a Canadian medical educator. She identifies deficits in three categories: knowledge, skills and attitude. When applied, they look like this.

Knowledge Deficits

Most medical students are fairly intelligent, high achievers. If there are knowledge deficits, it may be due to the distraction of competing personal, family or health concerns. If it truly is solely a knowledge problem, arranging for extra tutoring may help. These are typically the most easily addressed.

Skill Deficits

Communication skills are typically involved. These can be challenging for us to address in a community-based setting, as the learner who needs more practice will do so with our patients. Our concern for patient safety and care supersedes the educational needs of our learner. Closer supervision, monitoring and feedback may be required but may not always be possible within the confines of our clinical teaching practice. In a worst-case scenario, the practice will have to notify the program that they are not equipped to deal with this particular learner's needs. Before this, see if there is just not a good fit between preceptor and student. Would another clinical supervisor work more effectively with this learner?

Clinical exam skill weaknesses can generally be corrected with more supervised practice opportunities. Remember, we need to start where the learner is, not where we would like them to be. If the learner is motivated, we are generally willing to put in the extra effort such learners require. But a structured approach may be needed so that progress can be measured.

Attitude

Attitude is easily perceived, but difficult to completely describe and understand. One of the hallmarks of effective feedback is to try to focus on behaviors, which are somewhat more objective. This can be challenging with a learner with an attitude issue. Effective feedback also needs to be timely, so putting off the uncomfortable discussion will be counter-productive.

The initial tendency of many preceptors is that they are imagining things or just being too sensitive. Keep faith with your long-standing common sense and intuition, as well as the numerous previous students you have mentored. If you have a sense that something is just not right, you are in the best position to judge that. Knowing how to deal with it is another matter. We are unlikely to effect change in deeply rooted attitude misalignments, but calling someone on sloppiness, laziness or a perceived lack of interest may be the wake-up call they need.

A 1989 study by Hunt of 464 undergraduate preceptors at the University of Washington, examined the types and frequency of problems they faced. Students with non-cognitive issues (personality issues, affective disorder, substance abuse) posed the greatest challenge for preceptors, even though knowledge and skill deficits were more common.

GENERAL CONSIDERATIONS

Documenting the interventions and progress made is critical. If the learner is eventually not going to pass the final evaluation, they should not receive a passing grade at mid-term. If they mount an appeal against their unsatisfactory evaluation, a pass at mid-term is usually administratively inconsistent with a failing final grade.

Communicate with the program director and the learner early on. The program director may have suggestions for intervention or strategies for this particular leaner which have worked in the past.

Limit any potentially unsafe or worrisome patient-contact this learner might otherwise have. For example, letting a learner with poor communication skills follow-up counseling patients might be unwise and unfair to the patient. Leaving a weak resident on their own in the emergency department would be folly.

Identifying the Problem Learner

This may be an obviously late, clumsy or rude learner. Such focused deficits easily come to our attention. More commonly, our perception may begin more holistically with just a sense of unease. We should follow-up these feelings by asking our colleagues and office staff how they have found the learner's behavior. If a pattern exists, we need to document objective examples so that we can discuss them. It may be that the learner is unaware of it and agrees to attend to the issue. A follow-up discussion can be scheduled to see what progress has been made. If there is conflict around this, there may be more deep-seated issues for which an educational intervention alone may be inadequate.

We may not Succeed

The two ideal educational variables are the keen, hard-working learner and the skilled clinical teacher. In reality, we each lie on a continuum and hopefully the variables intersect in a healthy part of the bell curve. But not always. Let us assume the teacher has generally had very positive interactions with previous learners and they are otherwise on their game. We can point out and document problem issues and ask the learner's perspective. But we cannot "make the penny drop," or arrange an "epiphany." Community-based medical educators can note that what they see does not meet expected standards and explore alternative strategies. Like some of our patients, these learners will make their own choices and live with the consequences. If they are willing participants and agree to alternative strategies, much can be accomplished. But we must keep in mind that the problem belongs to the learner, not the preceptor in this scenario. We play a key role in identifying some of the obvious issues or their manifestations and are intimately involved in facilitating solutions, but the learner must be the main mover. The exception would be the preceptor–learner combination who just rub each other up the wrong way, due to wide differences in values or personality. In this case, changing preceptors may solve many of the problems.

Having an Approach

A community-based medical educator typically receives an evaluation form from their program. The program's approach to education and its standards can be distilled from these evaluation forms and they can serve as a bit of a map for beginning an educational assessment, even though it is not time for actually filling them out. Referring to these forms can help the preceptor know what to document in terms of deficiencies in an objective manner. But the program's philosophy behind these evaluations may not be completely obvious. We generally do better when we have a grasp of first principles. In theory, they are simple: document behaviors, discuss them with the learner and program director, attempt an "educational diagnosis," develop an educational plan and arrange close follow-up (*see* Table 8.1). Referrals and other services may also be needed. This may sound similar to our clinical practice, but the types of diagnoses and referrals are not those we encounter in patient care.

Table 8.1 Dealing with a Difficult Learner

Do	*Don't*
➤ Get assistance when you need it	➤ Assume your teaching is the cause
➤ Assume you are competent to identify poor performance	➤ Think the problem will solve itself
➤ Know that documentation must be very complete and specific	➤ Assume you will figure it all out
➤ Ask the learner's perspective	➤ Assume you will "solve" the learner's problems
➤ Attempt an "educational diagnosis"	➤ Attempt a "medical diagnosis" on the learner
➤ Agree upon a plan with deliverables	➤ Proceed without a documented plan
➤ Set scheduled follow-up discussions	➤ Be lax in observation and feedback

EDUCATIONAL DIAGNOSIS

Just as in practice where some patients tend to blame their problems on others (including their physician), some students may blame their difficulties on their preceptor. We are at a disadvantage: we feel somewhat inadequate because we are not "trained teachers." Resist this disadvantaged starting point. If all previous learners have thrived under your supervision, what is different now? The educational diagnosis may actually elude us as it sometimes does in clinical practice, but just as we do in primary care, we still must develop an approach to a given issue. Here, the correct set of "investigations" may not be as clear as many of our clinical scenarios. We may not come to a complete elaboration of the underlying issue, but we are capable of identifying and documenting substandard performance (*see* Table 8.2).

For example, poor concentration may be due to personal learner emotional issues, to unease in the present learning environment or to a language or actual learning disability. That is why it is important to be objective and, as non-judgmentally as possible, describe issues and seek the learner's perspective. If the learner agrees with the problem definition and co-operates, this may work out well. If they deny the identified behaviors are significant, or resist discussion or change, you are likely going to need to make a referral to an "educational specialist." That is likely to be the program director unless there is an identified program "troubleshooter."

The learner needs to know that their present performance is unacceptable or below par and not consistent with passing mid-term or final evaluations. They also need to be informed that you are seeking guidance from the program director. The director is able to review the past educational history and recognize this as a recurrent or new issue. They may or may not have concrete supervising suggestions, but at least they are now a part of the "education team."

Table 8.2 Educational Diagnosis and Treatment Planning

Learner difficulty	Identify problem behavior
	Get the learner's perspective
	Objectively state the behavior and its effect on staff and patients
	Identify the likely summative evaluation outcome
Educational diagnosis	*Referrals:* to another community preceptor and/or program director, program or support person
	Testing: could include: a trial with more supervision, role-modeling etc. The learner may agree to confidential medical and mental health assessment in another environment; actual reading/writing skill assessment
	Examination of *past history* will need involvement of the program director, and the learner must be made aware of any such communication; chronic or recurrent issues may need a program intervention perhaps beyond present community capabilities or a previous successful intervention can be re-instituted
Educational plan	The plan will be tailored to the educational "diagnosis," which may remain somewhat unclear, so behavior change needs to be routinely assessed and documented so that plans can be adjusted
Follow-up	Regular, predictable and documented follow-up is needed. More observed monitoring and feedback sessions are likely required and this will have an effect on preceptor and learner ability to continue with continue with routine volume of clinical workload

EDUCATIONAL PLAN

"In house" remedies of extra tutorial time spent on knowledge gaps are usually within our ability. Most preceptors will be more than willing to put in some extra time with a struggling student if the learner also puts in additional effort. Communication skills come to the surface through direct observation of the learner with a patient. Learners, who struggle with this, need to repeatedly see how it can be done well. This can be achieved by having the learner come in with the preceptor to see how they handle communication. Following each interview, the learner can discuss what they observed, essentially giving feedback to their preceptor. Role-playing in the patient role can also assist communication skill development and can include other learners. Then the learner can assume the physician role in role-playing and subsequently with patients, each time receiving direct observation and feedback.

We may need to set the bar at a different height. If it is clear that the learner will fail the rotation, is there still something to be gained? If we have the program's and the learner's agreement and it can be realistically and safely accomplished in a community-based setting, we can start where the learner is and move forward from there. That way an educational intervention has begun, even though it is clear they will need to repeat the rotation.

Attitudinal mismatches are challenging. We should ensure the learner has appropriate support for any mental health issues. Beyond that, monitoring problematic behaviors and expecting improvement after feedback is typically as far as we can go in a community-based rotation. The more problematic the behavior, the more program support and oversight of the learner will be needed.

SUMMARY

This is a relatively under-researched area of medical education. From what we do know, 5–10% of learners will encounter significant problems in their training. The majority can be assisted and ultimately remediated toward successful graduation.

The community-based medical educator will encounter learners in difficulty and our role is ideally placed to identify problem behaviors. A non-judgmental, documented highlighting of the issues is the first step. The learner's perspective should be sought. Early identification, documentation and contact with the program director are the key and basic elements of our responsibility.

Deficits in knowledge and skills are common, but pose less challenge to preceptors than non-cognitive (attitudinal) issues. Preceptors need to acknowledge their feeling that something is not quite right and follow that with seeking broad confidential input from colleagues and office staff and others. That way, the preceptor receives a "second opinion" around what they have noticed and they can share the emotionally draining load a challenging learner may present.

If patient and staff complaints have surfaced spontaneously, this may speak to a well-established problem. The learner needs to have feedback on these specific behaviors or incidents and be encouraged to give their perspective. The learner may react with some blaming, denial or anger. In concert with the program director, an educational plan is devised and careful follow-up organized. The preceptor should make notes on any meetings or discussions. Mid-term and final evaluations need to accurately reflect the situation. Traditionally, it seems we have not done well at this. A failing mid- and final-rotation evaluation may be the call to action the learner and program both need.

Meeting the learner's educational needs may not always be achievable in a particular community-based practice. The ultimate responsibility lies with the program, not the community-based preceptor. The few studies which have examined subsequent remediation interventions do show successful, although resource-intensive, outcomes. This needs to be a team effort, including the learner, program director and any other colleagues and services needed. Failing a learner on a given rotation may be a necessary but difficult educational undertaking. An organized approach may help neutralize some of the emotional impact this brings to both the learner and the teacher. It will be important that adequate support exists for both the learner and the teacher, so that each can move forward after the experience.

FURTHER READING

Association of American Medical Colleges, clinical evaluation project. *The Evaluation of Clinical Clerks: perceptions of clinical faculty.* Washington DC; 1983.

Carron P, Hutcheon M, Rothman A. Academic difficulty in postgraduate medical education; results of remedial programs at University of Toronto. *Ann RCPSC.* 2002; **35**(4): 232–7.

Dudel N, Marks M, Begehr G. Failure to fail: the perspectives of clinical supervisors. *Acad Med.* 2005; **80**: S84–7.

Earle L, Kelly L. Depression, anxiety and coping strategies in Ontario family medicine residents. *Can Fam Phys.* 2005; **51**: 243.

Hawkins C. The Failing Resident. In: *Teachers of Family Medicine Newsletter.* Mississauga ON, Canada: College of Family Physicians of Canada; Spring, 1997.

Hicks P, Cox S, Espey D, *et al.* To the point: medical education reviews – dealing with student difficulties in the clinical setting. *Am J Obstet Gynecol.* 2005; **193**: 1915–22.

Hunt D, Tonesk C, Yergan J, *et al.* Types of problem students encountered by clinical teachers on clerkships. *Med Educ.* 1989; **23**: 14–18.

Illot I. To fail or not to fail! A course for fieldwork educators. *Am J Occup Ther.* 1995; **49**: 251–5.

Langlois J, Thach S, Paulman P. Managing the difficult learning situation. *Fam Med.* 2000; **32**(5): 307–9.

Reamy B, Harman J. Residents in trouble; an in-depth assessment of the 25-year experience of a single family medicine residency. *Fam Med.* 2006; **38**(4): 252–7.

Roback H, Crowder M. Psychiatric resident dismissal: a national survey of training programs. *Am J Psych.* 1989; **146**: 96–8.

Sayer M, Sanitonge M, Evans D, *et al.* Support for students with academic difficulties. *Med Educ.* 2002; **36**: 643–50.

Steinert Y. The "problem" junior: whose problem is it? *BMJ.* 2008; **336**: 150–3.

Steinert Y, Levitt C. Working with the "problem" resident: guidelines for definition and intervention. *Fam Med.* 1993: **25**: 627–32.

Yao D, Wright S. National survey of internal medicine residency program directors regarding problem residents. *JAMA.* 2000; **284**(9): 1099–104.

9

Setting up a Teaching Practice

Lucie Walters

INTRODUCTION

At some point, the majority of doctors working in community practice will be approached to supervise medical students in their practice or to increase their teaching load. This chapter outlines the factors affecting the decision to teach medical students and highlights the strategic importance of precepting medical students in community practice for development of a sustainable medical workforce. Tips for formalizing the leadership and financial model within the practice are considered, together with the organization of practice systems to reward teaching and learning.

MAKING THE DECISION

Business Decisions

The decision to take students is usually both a personal one and a collective business decision, as community practice is often a shared or group practice with a finite capacity to service patients and generate an income. Decisions are made in this context. Since income is a part of the equation, some models of reimbursement may be perceived as better lending themselves to teaching. But, it can work in most scenarios. The independent fee for a service physician will be decided on their own, while those in group or managed-care practices will have additional inputs into developing a teaching practice.

Perceived Disadvantages

Time and productivity are the most frequent concerns raised in regard to clinical teaching in community practice. There is conflicting evidence regarding the impact of clinical teaching on time. Some preceptor studies report an average additional 27–120 minutes per day; however, 20–40% of doctors in these studies reported no increase in time. Productivity studies, measuring patients seen and income generated, have similar variation in evidence, with from zero to five fewer patients per day. These contradictory study results are partly caused by study method, with greater negative impact being found in studies which relied on retrospective self-reporting when compared with logs, diaries and prospective objective measurements. This is consistent with Nelson's 1975 finding that clinicians are unable to accurately recollect their own activities. Solo practitioners are more likely to report teaching taking extra time, while fee-for-service physicians express more concerns about productivity. These studies show that impacts on one's practice are also dependent on type of student placement and how students are managed in the practice, and we will look at these considerations.

Recent Australian studies have shown that where the learner has access to their own consulting room to see patients before being joined by the GP (parallel consulting), there is no increase in consultation time. The total time of teaching and seeing patients was also unaffected by GP experience in teaching, GP reported interest in teaching, student feedback on effectiveness of teaching, or length of student attachment (after the first four weeks). If the student had their own room, Australian rural physicians saw the same number of patients per day and had an increase of only 10 minutes per day in non-patient contact time. The supervision of a medical student in this study was time neutral, exclusive of any end-of-day debriefing or discussion topics which may arise. Postgraduate learners, registrars or residents, will have often seen patients on their own during the day. They will require a chart review of each patient seen and their management approved by the clinical supervisor. This extra time will typically be more than offset by the patient billing they can generate in most settings.

Another frequently raised concern regarding clinical teaching is the discomfort some doctors feel when being scrutinized by a student. This perception can be ameliorated considerably by reframing clinical precepting as facilitating student learning, rather than teaching. Clinicians are not expected to be the fount of all clinical knowledge, but rather provide students and junior doctors with opportunities to exercise and test their own knowledge, so identifying their gaps and motivating them to learn further.

Benefits

There are many: variety from typical daily patient care – the spice of a teaching practice. Having learners in our practice also supplies us with: intellectual stimulation; the opportunity to evaluate one's own approach and to learn from the students who may be more up-to-date; confidence and recognition for expertise and satisfaction from sharing and giving back to the profession. One of the key issues for those who practice in underserviced areas is that exposing learners to your community is one of the strategic ways of recruiting new physicians to your practice.

Clinical placements allow students to gradually develop identities as novice members of specific interest groups within the medical profession. Year-long rural community placements have been shown to influence students' future career choices: these students were 19 times more likely to choose rural practice than their tertiary-hospital-based peers, after correcting for age and rural background. Their clinical teachers are also more likely to remain in the community themselves as the career variation within community practice is an effective retention tool for rural doctors.

LEADERSHIP AND FINANCIAL CONSIDERATIONS

Once a commitment is made by a community practice to proceed with teaching medical students, it is important to formalize who is primarily responsible for clinical teaching, how supervised consulting sessions will be distributed between the doctors in the practice and how any financial remuneration will be divided. Typically, funds will be supplied per student, per time allotment. If students are generally shared and moved around in a practice, the funds can be jointly kept and used to reduce overhead costs or fund other group benefits.

Different models exist, from equal distribution, to distribution based on the contribution made by each doctor to student supervision and teaching. If the organizing physician is not centrally remunerated, then their time needs to be supported by these funds.

UNIVERSITY CONTRACT/AGREEMENT

Formal agreements or contracts with a University or Medical School exist in many countries. These can be with individual physicians or clinics, groups or hospitals. Elective students can often be accommodated into most practices, but mandatory core rotations bring a higher level of educational responsibility and reporting. If a formal agreement is required, it is important to ensure all parties are clear about their roles and responsibilities, and that expectations are explicit – particularly regarding how many learners will be accepted at one time.

An effective agreement should outline: what services the teaching clinician or practice is expected to provide, how the university will support the practice and clinical teachers, and remuneration associated with this agreement. Many agreements also include the expectations of medical students on placement and the learning and evaluation expectations. University support may include: recognition through academic status or personal certificate or practice signage, infrastructure support or rental payments, professional indemnity and public liability insurance, professional development, remediation of underperforming medical students. Other less common, but highly valued supports, include: involving GP supervisors in the selection of students for placement in their region or practice, and further engagement in academic medicine, for example, through research bursaries or scholarships. All these perks are balanced by the expectations of the practice's contribution to clinical teaching. Universities may be explicit about the range of clinic responsibilities, including, provision of student orientation, student access to facilities including consulting room space and to an area with internet access for private study. Clinical supervisors may also be expected to provide students with: opportunities to actively participate in patient care under supervision, regular formal tutorials or teaching sessions, timely and accurate student assessments and reports, and participation in university meetings and professional development to remain up-to-date with curriculum expectations.

As well as ensuring an explicit understanding of the role of each party in medical student placements, these agreements also provide the opportunity for practices to understand the educational responsibilities they are taking on, and seek advice regarding the legal risk inherent and the strategies recommended to ensure that the practice risk-manages the implications of a student failing to meet the assessment requirements of the medical course.

Once these issues are understood and the partnership is comfortable with the requirements for student supervision, it is time to organize the logistics of student placements. Arranging logistics such as student travel and accommodation is assumed to be the responsibility of the university.

HOW TO SET UP AN OFFICE

Parallel consulting, where medical students see a patient prior to the clinician joining the consultation provides students with an active role in the clinical context, without impacting on the time spent by doctors with each patient. There may be times when clinic rooms are too small, where the student follows the preceptor along for consultations. This is very useful for short periods, as we all benefit from comparing our practice with peers or experts; however, it is obviously counter-productive as the only experience for learners at any level. Like every member of staff, students require access to facilities and amenities appropriate to the occupational health and safety of their role. As medical students on placement, they will be required to consolidate their clinical experience through studying the relevant presentations and clinical treatment options. Student study space is required in order that students do not interfere with the patient care activities of other clinic staff, or impact on patient flow, particularly patient waiting times.

BOOKING STUDENT APPOINTMENTS

Assuming that most practice booking systems allow doctors to choose appointment times and designate appointments for specific purposes, these tools can be used to organize student appointments. If space is available for students to see patients, prior to being joined by the family physician, appointment times can be altered to reduce patient waiting times. We outline here the "parallel booking system" which can be very time efficient.

Figure 9.1 illustrates a standard booking sheet where Dr. Jones has a solo consulting session seeing patients every 15 minutes. Figure 9.2 illustrates a student consulting session. Every 30 minutes, two patients commence appointment. Patient "1" has a 15-minute appointment with Dr. Jones in Room 1, and is unlikely to have student involvement. Meanwhile, Patient "2" sees the student in Room 2 for 15 minutes before being joined by Dr. Jones for the second half of their 30-minute student appointment. This booking schedule allows Dr. Jones to continue to see patients every 15 minutes (alternating solo consultations with precepting consultations) and minimizes disruptions to patient flow.

0900	Patient 1	Room 1
0915	Patient 2	Room 1
0930	Patient 3	Room 1
0945	Patient 4	Room 1

Figure 9.1 Dr. Jones' Usual Booking Sheet

0900	Patient 1	Room 1
0915	Patient 2 – Designated student appointment	Room 2
0930	Patient 3	Room 1
0945	Patient 4 – Designated student appointment	Room 2

Figure 9.2 Dr. Jones' Student Consulting Session

PATIENT CONSENT

Explicit patient consent to see learners is an essential part of ethical practice. If a learner is a resident, they have an educational license and can have patients booked directly with them. The patient needs to be told that they are seeing a resident, or junior doctor, and under whose supervision they function. "I can book you in with Dr. Smith's resident and they will be checking in with Dr. Smith about your treatment." Generally, such newly independent physicians should be booked no more than every 20 minutes. This scheduling may need to be decreased at first, but toward the end of their training, challenging them with a near-full caseload in the office is useful in their training. Patients quickly learn that such junior doctors are interested, keen and up-to-date in addressing their needs.

Consent for medical students' involvement in patient care must also be explicit and systematized with the practice. Signs in the waiting room and reception desk should state that this is a teaching practice and, if possible, identify learners currently in the practice by name and photo.

If using the parallel booking system, appointment staff can specifically offer designated student appointments and clarify that they will be joined by the attending physician part-way through the 30-minute consultation. The patient should have an opportunity to decline seeing a medical student. This can be done in various ways via the intercession of the receptionist or clinic nurse, but should not rely on the patient having to directly confront the student. This may still sometimes happen despite our best intentions. It is important to reassure the patient that it is their choice and not a problem, but also to advise the student not to take this important patient decision personally.

Clearly, the need to inform and seek explicit consent increases as the invasiveness or personal nature of the interaction does. A patient may well consent to discussing their issue with a student, but may prefer their regular physician to perform an internal or rectal exam.

ORIENTATION OF STUDENTS

Orientation of students can be somewhat neglected in a busy practice when clinicians and staff are time-poor, particularly if there is a high turnover of students. It is an important preventative strategy to minimize the risk of misunderstandings and maximize the capacity for students to feel welcome and be able to contribute meaningfully to clinical care.

Suggested content for student orientation includes: introductions to key staff including, whoever the students should go to for clinical issues, administrative matters and occupational health and safety issues. It is helpful for students to have a booklet or intranet site with staff names and photos, so they can quickly call staff by name and understand their roles within the practice.

Many universities now provide students with sessions on their code of practice and legislative requirements for clinical placements such as: patient confidentiality, patient consent, mandatory reporting, and antidiscrimination obligations. It may be helpful for the practice to ask for a written document from the medical school confirming students are covered by indemnity insurance and that students understand and have committed to work within the relevant legislation on clinical placement. The hospital or practice may request a letter of good standing from the host university. They have the right to know if any serious problems have been encountered in the past with this learner. Some programs have policies against such potentially prejudicial "forward feeding." This will need to be clarified with each host university.

Orientation to the practice can then focus on context-specific expectations such as dress and behavior standards, use of medical equipment, office and internet resources and how the morning tea roster works. Orientation is also the time for the primary supervisor to find out the student's self-assessment of their strengths and weaknesses, agree on some learning objectives and plan formative and summative feedback, in line with the placement requirements. It is helpful to state a caveat up front such as "I will arrange to provide you with feedback more frequently, if I have any concerns." More on this topic has been addressed in the chapters on contracting, monitoring and feedback (*see* Chapters 2, 3 and 4 respectively).

INTEGRATING STUDENTS INTO CORE BUSINESS

Community practices are complex adaptive systems, which are constantly changing and adapting. It is important that the process of having students in the practice becomes automatic. This can be systematized by adopting procedures and policies for orientation, student appointments, patient consent, student teaching and learning and the provision of feedback. It is important that this systematization extends to practice evaluation. Practice surveys should ask patients about their experience with students. Staff meetings and clinical meetings should also include students as a regular agenda item. Finally, students should be offered an opportunity to provide feedback at the end of their placement, as part of the information contributing to a continuous quality improvement cycle.

SUMMARY

Becoming a teaching practice is a feather in the cap of any practice. With an increased sense of professional self-worth comes a doable educational role for us. Developing predictability for patients, staff, learners and the clinical teachers comes in time with a bit of effort. For most of us, combining an educational role with our clinical work will immensely enhance our careers.

FURTHER READING

Baldor R, Brooks W, Warfield M, *et al.* A survey of primary care physicians' perception and needs regarding the precepting of medical students in their offices. *Med Educ.* 2001; **35**(8): 714–15.

Bell J, Frey D. Survey shows impacts of students in preceptors' offices. *Fam Med.* 1998; **30**(2): 82.

Nelson E, Jacobs A, Breer P. A study of the validity of the task inventory method of job analysis. *Med Care*. 1975; **13**(2): 104–113.

Vinson D, Paden C. The effect of teaching medical students on private practitioners' workloads. *Acad Med*. 1994; **69**: 237–8.

Walters L, Worley P, Prideaux D, *et al*. Do consultations in rural general practice take more time when practitioners are precepting medical students? *Med Educ*. 2008; **42**: 69–73.

Walters L. *How and Why Rural General Practitioners Commit the Time to Precept Medical Students*. Adelaide: Flinders University; 2009.

Walters L, Worley P, Greenhill J. Demonstrating the value of longitudinal integrated placements for GP preceptors. *Med Educ*. 2011, in press.

Wirth P, Kahn L, Perkoff G. Comparability of two methods of time and motion study used in a clinical setting: work sampling and continuous observation. *Med Care*. 1997; **15**(11): 953–60.

10

Culture in Medicine

Len Kelly

Culture and medicine keep company in many ways and include the patient, learner, teacher and their profession. The predominant reference to culture in the healthcare delivery literature appropriately highlights patient care (cultural safety): how physicians can understand and effectively treat patients of another culture. A subset of this is how we teach this skill, typically called cultural competence, to our learners. The third theme is the result of the medical migration of our trainees. How can medical educators train learners of another culture to function as fully effective clinicians in our culture? How do we travel the educational and interpersonal space between the clinical teacher and learner of different cultures? Superimposed on these ethnic challenges is the perspective of medicine itself as a socialization process, an enculturation (*see* Table 10.1).

Table 10.1 Cultural Presence in Medicine

➤ Cultural safety: patients feel safe and cultural issues are part of care planning
➤ Cultural competence: training to acknowledge the patient–caregiver cultural gap
➤ Cross-cultural trainees: education of students from another culture
➤ Enculturation: adoption of professional values, attitudes and behavior

These first three themes share part of the simple, but often circuitous journey, from "them" to "us." All have the common requirement of a degree of self-awareness: an understanding of one's own personal biases and cultural imperatives. These are assumptions for us, but pose potential barriers for others. Underlying these characterizations of culture-as-ethnicity is the sociological perspective of the profession of medicine as its own culture. This is sometimes referenced in the medical education literature as a "hidden curriculum," a process where many important attributes of the profession are passed from teacher to learner outside of the classroom.

CULTURAL SAFETY OF PATIENTS

Patient safety is a well-established medical concept with established hospital practices: infection control surveillance, incident reporting, patient surveys. Cultural safety is an emerging concept and is somewhat analogous to learner safety, a concept we introduce here. The idea of cultural safety first emerged in New Zealand nursing education in the late 1980s. It developed as a response to the inequalities experienced by minorities in relation to their interactions with healthcare professionals with whom there was both a power and dominant culture differential. Patients who are culturally or ethnically different from the mainstream are at higher risk of experiencing adverse health events considered preventable if it were not for language or cultural differences.

The concept of cultural safety, which was originally used in the context of interactions between different racial or ethnic groups, has been expanded by some, to be applicable in any clinical interaction between individuals with different worldviews. Cultural safety is predicated on the understanding that a caregiver's own culture, and assumptions, impact the manner in which a clinical encounter is played out and therefore impacts the patient's care. The burden of cultural adaptation that results when intercultural interactions occur should be relieved from the patient whenever possible.

Cultural safety is essential for clinical safety: minimizing risk and providing a safe healing environment. Cultural safety educators aim to impart the understanding that past and present socio-political processes are intrinsically connected to contemporary health and social issues. Knowledge of cultural differences (cultural awareness) is only the first step in the process diagrammed below. Earlier discussions of cross-cultural awareness often stalled at oversimplification and stereotyping that focused on the differences between cultures. Cultural safety educators now focus on the differences between how various cultures are treated and on self-awareness. At the level of the individual, cultural competence focuses on patient-centered care, which improves care regardless of nationality, culture, age, gender or religious beliefs.

The simplest analysis of cultural safety is seen graphically in a hospital-based cultural safety initiative at the Meno Ya Win Health Centre in Sioux Lookout, Ontario, where over 80% of patients are North American First Nations. The hospital developed a conceptual overview called the Continuum of Cross Cultural Client Safety (see Figure 10.1). Language, which is the tip of the attitudinal iceberg, often alerts us to the potential of a "them and us" scenario. It can reference the presence of thoughts and attitudes which lie below the surface. A true understanding of the imbalances in a caregiver–patient dynamic requires the caregiver to engage in a process of self-reflection in which one's own culture and assumptions are understood and recognized. This attitude of "cultural humility" requires an enduring commitment to self-evaluation and self-critique by the caregiver. At Meno Ya Win, the patients' cultural values are factored into their care plan. Additionally, hospital staff attend cultural work-shops which use role-playing and storytelling to mitigate the distance different languages and beliefs bring. The objective is to move from thinking of patients who are of a different culture as "them" to a more inclusive "us."

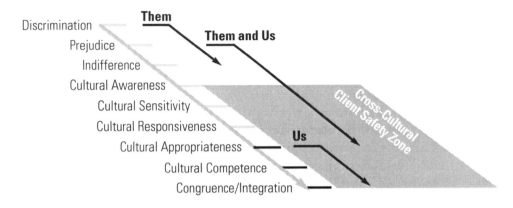

Adapted with permission from Walker and Cromarty, 2006 Sioux Lookout, Meno Ya Win Health Centre

Figure 10.1 Continuum of Cultural Safety

Cultural safety therefore entails a degree of self-examination and reflection by the clinician. It also takes time. In a qualitative study of experienced clinicians deal-ing with First Nations patient populations in Canada, Kelly outlined a process of increasing comfort with silence, less eye contact and a more indirect approach to topics of discussion. The process usually took the clinician between 3 and 5 years working in specific cross-cultural settings. This study described the natural cultural adaptation process physicians underwent if they stayed in the field of cross-cultural care, with changes in their attitudes and behavior. Physicians show their respect by learning some of their patients' language. Healthcare institutions can do the same by providing training and funding for medical translation services where needed, as these staff often take on the unrecognized additional role of cultural navigator for patients. Cultural advisory groups also have a role to play in the development of institutional policy when they function in bicultural settings.

It is difficult to understand the cultural starting point for many patients of another culture. Their health literacy (how and what they know about their own and their family's health) and medical literacy (how the healthcare system func-tions) will be largely implicit and even attitudinal. It is only with time and open-ness that a physician or institution can access this initial patient perspective.

TEACHING CULTURAL COMPETENCE

Being able to deal with patients of another culture has now become a part of the accreditation of North American medical undergraduate and residency programs. The North American Liaison Committee of Medical Education (LCME) includes cultural competence as a part of professionalism. Subsequently, many programs have developed initiatives at developing this cross-cultural communication skill set. They commonly entail a series of educational sessions on the beliefs and practices of specific cultures the learner might encounter which are the first steps along the continuum of cultural competence. At the other end of the educational spectrum are leading-edge initiatives in clearly bicultural social environments. The Northern Ontario School of Medicine in Canada not only has didactic and case-based learning around First Nations healthcare, it also has a mandatory 1-month undergraduate placement in a remote Aboriginal community. These community-based experiences are at the invitation of the health director of each community and expose medical students to the reality of life and medical care challenges in remote, and often impoverished, communities.

In multicultural urban-based programs, learning multicultural caregiving requires developing a patient-centeredness to allow for, as yet, unencountered cultural presentations. These programs will by necessity focus on knowledge of diverse cultures and communication skills, along with some required physician focus on self-awareness.

An often unrecognized perspective is the "institutional ethos" about how those of other cultures are treated. Institutional ethos, as influenced by differences in language and race, will have an effect on teaching cultural competence in learners. If there is good correlation between the learning content, behavior modeling and institutional environment, learners will avoid the dissonance pres-

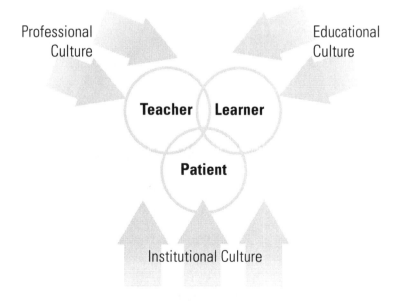

Figure 10.2 Cultural Influences on Medical Care and Education

ent when they are in conflict, and have to navigate often dissimilar standards. This is akin to the "hidden curriculum" associated with medical educational programs, with unspoken but real sub-cultural imperatives that lead behavior and thinking within a given work and learning environment. Institutional ethos is resistant to overt description and acknowledgement (*see* Figure 10.2).

CROSS-CULTURAL LEARNER SAFETY

There are parallels between the delivery of appropriate cross-cultural patient care and the adjustment required of the educational system to accommodate the medical migration of trainees from other cultures and medical systems. Adjusting to a new and typically dominant culture is stressful. Learning is stressful. Doing both simultaneously without much of a safety net is the lot of many international medical learners.

We know that learning environments need to be supportive. Learners of another culture will spend a lot of energy adapting. There may even be cultural implications to an institution's basic approach to education. Problem-based learning, established at McMaster University in the 1980s, involves active student participation and group learning. This may not be a good fit for Asian communication styles, which exhibit respectful cultural reticence toward disputing another's opinion. It may also be at cultural odds with the North American First Nations communication style of indirect communication and "non-interference." These differences might need specific cultural supports rendered by clinical teachers of the same culture or additional cross-cultural training for teachers and students. Similar to patient-centeredness, our optimal approach for learner safety is "student-centeredness."

Learners who experience suboptimal learning safety are more likely to lose their own ability to treat patients optimally. A Belgian medical student focus group study by Bombeke *et al* in 2010 identified the student–supervisor relationship as the key to learning patient-centeredness. Not only did a supportive learning environment enhance students' self-development, it facilitated the direct transmission of patient-centered skills, knowledge and attitudes. This was primarily accomplished through the role-modeling by the clinical teacher, treating both the student and the patient "as-person." Clearly our modern medical learning environment is complex. Aside from ethnic culture, does medical training impose a further sociological sub-culture with a hidden curriculum?

MEDICAL PROFESSION AS CULTURE

We learn a lot of information and skills during our medical training. We also learn how to think and act like a physician. The sub-culture of medicine becomes apparent as students begin their work in clinical settings, where they are exposed to the role models who practice and "not just teach" medicine. The process most apparently begins when students hit the wards, and this may include rotations with community-based teachers.

Students learn in both the classroom and coffee room. The curricula are different, sometimes even antithetical. The term "hidden curriculum" was first used in medical education in 1994 by Hafferty, an American sociologist, who documented the acquisition of professional identity which occurred outside the classroom. At the time, medical programs were instituting ethics courses in response to the public perception of an erosion of the character of physicians. The assumption was that learning more about ethics would address the problem. Hafferty pointed out that ethics courses did not take place in an ethically neutral environment. He described that a large part of learning medicine took place in the hallways more than in the classroom, through this hidden curriculum. This enculturation process encouraged emotional detachment and the objectification of patients. Medical students were learning and adopting the values, attitudes and behaviors of their profession's leaders, with both negative and positive components.

In a 2010 qualitative study, Gaufberg characterized the hidden curriculum as including: the decline of idealism, the prominence of hierarchy, emotional suppression and patient objectification; but all was not negative. This study of 30 American clinical clerks also demonstrated the importance of human connections for the student and the patient, and the emergence of a sense of accountability and duty toward patient care and learning. The 2006 Belgium medical student study found that a supportive student–supervisor relationship could temper negative influences and was the key to learning patient-centered care.

Our role-modeling as clinical teachers about key issues of power and respect may be more influential than what (little) we know about the immune system, for example. The oral tradition of jokes and anecdotes are powerful moderators of this cultural process. Like all coping strategies, they are a mixed bag that promotes survival in the learning and practicing environment established by our preceptors.

SUMMARY

Cultural humility begins at home. If we are to understand the hurdles another culture must go through or over to accommodate (or assimilate) to our own, we will need a good degree of self-awareness, patience and perhaps educational interventions for us and our learner. This is a tall order for a busy clinician and they will need program support for the extra time and energy this may require through faculty development and beyond.

Foreign medical graduates have to cope with these multiple agendas while they interpret the subtle cues of medical communication and humor. Imagine yourself a cultural neophyte in that environment. Welcome to the doctors' lounge! Try to start your day in both a new culture and an almost impenetrable subculture and see if the most relaxing part of your day doesn't begin until you are actually dealing with just patients! In the following chapter, Wearne and associates will discuss facilitating the effective training of these international medical graduates.

FURTHER READING

Anderson C. Cultural competency (also known as nursing competency). *Nurs Outlook.* 2002; **50**:175.

Bischoff A. *Caring for Migrant and Minority Patients in European Hospitals: a review of effective interventions.* Vienna: Migrant Friendly Hospitals; 2003.

Bombeke K, Symons L, Debaene L, *et al.* Help, I'm losing patient centeredness! Experiences of medical students and teachers. *Med Educ.* 2010; **44**(7): 662–73.

Brant C. Native ethics and rules of behaviour. *Can J Psych.* 1990; **35**: 534–9.

Choon-Eng Gwee M. Globalization of problem based learning: cross-cultural implications. *Kaohsiung J Med Sci.* 2008; **24**(3): S14–22.

Dogra N, Reitmanova S, Carter-Pokras O. Twelve tips for teaching diversity and embedding it in the medical curriculum. *Med Teach.* 2009; **31**: 990–3.

Gaufberg E, Batalden M, Sands R. The hidden curriculum: what can we learn from third year medical student narrative reflections? *Acad Med.* 2010; **85**(11): 1709–16.

Guilfoyle J, Kelly L, St Pierre-Hansen N. Prejudice in medicine. *Can Fam Phys.* 2008; **54**(11): 1511–13.

Hafferty K, Franks R. The hidden curriculum, ethics teaching and the structure of medical education. *Acad Med.* 1994; **69**(11): 861–71.

Hauer K, Boscardin C, Gesundheit N, *et al.* Impact of student ethnicity and patient-centeredness on communication skills performance. *Med Educ.* 2010; **44**(7): 653–61.

Hoff T, Pohl H, Bartfield J. Creating a learning environment to produce competent residents: the roles of culture and context. *Acad Med.* 2004; **79**(6): 532–9.

Kelly L, Brown J. Listening to native patients. *Can Fam Phy.* 2002; **48**: 1645–52.

Kuper A, D'Eon M. Rethinking the basis of medical knowledge. *Med Educ.* 2011; **45**: 36–43.

Lempp H, Seale C. The hidden curriculum in undergraduate medical education: qualitative study of medical students' perceptions of teaching. *BMJ.* 2004; **329**: 770–3.

Murray-Garcia J, Garcia J. The institutional context of multicultural education: what is your institutional curriculum? *Acad Med.* 2008; **83**(7): 646–52.

National Aboriginal Health Organization (NAHO). *Cultural Competency and Safety: A guide for healthcare administrators, providers and educators.* Ottawa: NAHO; 2008.

Paasche-Orlow M. The ethics of cultural competence. *J Med Educ.* 2004; **79**(4): 347–50.

Ramsden I. Equalizing the partnership. *NZ Nurs J.* 1989; **82**(2): 2.

Ramsden I, Spoonley P. The cultural safety debate in nursing education in Aotearoa. *NZ Ann Rev Educ.* 1993; **3**: 161–74.

Smye V, Browne A. 'Cultural safety' and the analysis of health policy affecting Aboriginal people. *Nurs Res.* 2002; **9**(3): 42–56.

Walker R, Cromarty H, Kelly L, *et al.* Achieving cultural safety in aboriginal health services: implementation of a cross-cultural safety model in a hospital setting. *Diversity in Health and Care.* 2009: **6**(1): 11–22.

11

Teaching International Medical Graduates

Susan Wearne, Sandy Wells, Anna MacLeod and Blye Frank

Two concurrent social trends are impacting the provision of medical education and healthcare in developed countries. The first is the increasing proportion of internationally educated healthcare practitioners, International Medical Graduates (IMGs), in our healthcare workforce. Recent estimates suggest that 25% of practicing physicians in North America are graduates of international medical schools, as are 50% of physicians in rural Australia. Many of these trainees report feeling discrimination and bias when transferring their skills to their new context. The second is the increasing, and shifting, cultural diversity of the patients being served in both rural and urban settings, coupled with the recognition that many historically marginalized groups continue to receive inadequate healthcare. Both trends have significant implications for those who teach and license healthcare practitioners. Not only do teachers of IMGs need to discover and teach to the different needs and strengths of learners from different social and medical traditions, but they must also prepare these various healthcare workers to address the healthcare diversity in their new context.

ORIENTATION
Leaving Home and Starting Out
A medical degree is a form of international currency and the worldwide shortage of physicians has created unprecedented opportunities for medical migration. Doctors respond to differing push and pull factors as they leave their home country and work in a new location. A minority migrate to serve in less well resourced areas or in aid work, but many migrate hoping for improved circumstances only to find that the jobs they are offered are in areas where home grown physicians choose not to work. The decision to leave home is a big one and requires considerable determination and organization – it is

rare for this to be guilt- or stress-free. As a result, medical migrants and their families often arrive bearing a mix of emotions, expectations, experience and exhaustion.

Welcoming International Medical Graduates

Relationships and first impressions do matter. The sooner, and more practical, your welcome, the better your relationship will be. It can be hard to know where to start with orientation and teaching, and Maslow's hierarchy of needs provides a useful framework for deciding: basic needs come first, followed by social needs. Some IMGs describe being met off their international flight and taken to their short-term accommodation with a starter box of food provided. They found this a memorable, practical demonstration of support. As the clinical supervisor, you may need to extend your usual teaching role to being tour guide and community aide, advising on schools, shopping, churches or mosques.

It is a justifiable investment to allow the newly arrived physician to use the work phone to reassure their family back home that they have arrived safely. Next are their safety requirements, which include arranging longer-term accommodation, meeting family needs, ensuring access to healthcare and establishing communication links. Learning how to care for a house and to cook may be a challenge for doctors who have always had servants in their home country. Setting up bank accounts, internet access and mobile phones in a new country can be hard, as migrants have no prior credit rating, let alone an understanding of the bureaucratic phrases and forms in a foreign language. Hopefully, effective infrastructure has been established in your program's central administration, to assist with these issues before the resident arrives in your practice.

Use your expertise in establishing rapport to find out about the IMG you will be supervising. A world atlas can be a starting point to have them tell you about their home country, their training, language, prior work experience and family. Google Earth might allow the IMG to show you their home village, town or city.

Culture and Context

Some say that "a doctor is a doctor." Well, yes and a loud NO. Medicine is a socio-cultural profession. Each of us has our own way of experiencing the world, illness and healing. Often the extent of these differences only becomes overt when traveling or working in a new country. Coupled with that can be a certainty or ethnocentricity that our way of doing something is correct, which creates considerable potential for conflict when people from different cultures work together. Some IMGs report that it is disorienting to be valued for your skills and then be told you are wrong!

Establishing Goals: is this Rotation a Stepping Stone or a Destination?

Do not assume that all those training to be GPs, want to be GPs. Just because we think this is your profession of choice, does not mean that perspective is shared. So gently ask the IMG what their short-term and then longer-term goals are. If GP training is their aim, it is worth confirming how your country perceives this role, and explore how this might differ from the expectations and perceptions in their home country. In particular, the doctor–patient partnership approach to practice in many Western countries can be uncomfortable or even a shock to doctors inculcated with the idea of doctors as authoritarian dispensers of pills and advice.

Getting Started

Orientation for IMGs should include more information about the wider health system, including details on funding arrangements and the expected patterns of use of specialists, nursing and allied health staff. A deliberate introduction, seeing patients with a clinical supervisor initially, and then seeing a small number of patients with ready access to supervision, will establish a solid foundation that easily repays the time and effort made. Expecting an IMG to quickly take a full clinical load may cause them to struggle and not reach their full potential in your practice.

Hospital and Other Community Staff

Introducing an IMG to the main hospital staff and giving guidance on how the local system operates is essential. The role of community staff such as physiotherapists and occupational therapists may be best learned by spending time watching them in practice. Investing time in visiting the local pharmacy and developing working relationships with the pharmacists is also invaluable.

In-house Meetings and Interdisciplinary Rounds

Regular practice meetings are an opportunity for foreign graduate learners to see how physicians interact and discuss cases. Working in an atmosphere where everyone can ask questions is a great help for the IMGs to feel encouraged to seek help, and learn the different roles of the healthcare team.

Online Resources

The internet provides opportunities for doctors in even the remotest areas to access a wealth of educational resources, but the quality varies greatly. Some advertising is "sold" as being educational. Bookmark your suggested sites, including a reputable source for drug information.

In-house Library

Choosing books can be personal, but useful recommendations for IMGs would include:

➤ General practice textbook
➤ General medical textbook
➤ Dermatology textbook plus an atlas of local skin conditions
➤ Text on women's health and contraception
➤ Text on requesting and interpreting laboratory results
➤ Copies of local and national guidelines
➤ Formulary
➤ Medical dictionary
➤ Slang dictionary!

(Some of these may be made available online)

Intimate Clinical Examinations

These merit special attention. Ideally, IMGs will have an opportunity to observe your practice and the appropriate use of chaperones, physical dexterity and the professional, empathic approach to the patient. Subsequent direct observation will provide an opportunity to watch your IMG perform these examinations and ensure their skills are appropriate.

Regular Frequent Feedback

As mentioned above, feedback is a vital component of medical education, but how this is given and received will vary in different cultures. Clearly explain the role and use of feedback and make an effort to give it early and regularly so that it becomes a habit. It can be difficult to provide and receive negative feedback, so consider your starting point carefully. Separate your role as the primary clinical supervisor of the IMG and the administrative role of the residency program director. These two people will need to communicate regularly but the different roles are more effectively enacted if clearly demarcated.

COMMON PROBLEMS FOR INTERNATIONAL MEDICAL GRADUATES

"Saving Face"

It can be difficult for some IMGs to acknowledge a knowledge deficit because of their cultural need/expectation of "saving face." The suggestions above of affirming and respecting what is known can help preserve someone's dignity so that admitting gaps is less psychologically risky. Make it clear that not knowing everything is a universal experience for GPs, and role-model looking things up or asking for assistance.

If, despite the evidence from objective assessments, an IMG is still reluctant to acknowledge knowledge gaps, more confronting methods such as a mock-exam may be necessary. Sometimes, it has taken a failure in a real exam to change a person's confidence and differing perception of competence. Your role is to stand back and watch carefully and then sensitively step back in and offer support for the repeat exam.

Use of Language

IMGs are usually required to take language proficiency tests prior to starting, but patients can still find it difficult to understand a different accent. Some IMGs work with speech therapists to prevent miscommunication. For IMGs with English as a second or third language, it is helpful to point out the difference between medical English and colloquial English. The colloquial use of a word, such as diarrhea, can have many more meanings than the medical English. There is a need for constant checking of understanding. Similarly, it can take a while to grasp the concept that just because a word is English does not mean that it is understood by all English speakers.

Writing

Another issue is handwriting. While much of medical practice relies on computers, some clinical notes and exams are handwritten. Consider asking the IMG to do a written test to ensure their writing is legible. There is a risk of this sounding patronizing, but the greater risk is someone failing an exam because the examiner could not read their otherwise excellent answers.

"Just Tell Me What To Do"

The differing education systems in many countries can create learners who expect to be told what, when and how to learn. Some IMGs may feel more comfortable receiving a mini-lecture on a given topic rather than being asked to share or discuss their views. When they are offered the chance to run educational sessions, some may also choose to deliver a lecture. It is best to resist the lecture model and redirect those who prefer this style to some of the online lectures. Trying to change an ingrained learning style while the learner is facing so many other challenges could create more stress than the desired professional development.

ASSESSMENT

There is a common presumption that IMGs' learning needs will center on language, culture and the new health system. This is often true, but a systematic approach to assessing learning needs and strengths is needed (*see* Table 11.1). It is worth finding out about the learner's specific interests and past experiences, so that any educational relationship is based on mutuality rather than uni-directionality. An international graduate physician who has been an ophthalmologist can give you updates on eye exam skills; a rehabilitation physician may inform your options for pain management and an ex-neurosurgeon can turn conducting a cranial nerve examination into an art form. Advertise their language skills so that patients who speak the same language in your community can consult with them. Creating a forum where

Table 11.1 Examples of Learning Needs Identified in Teaching IMGs

Basic sciences	Limited understanding of pathophysiology made it difficult to predict and explain disease process to patients
Biomedical understanding of illness	IMG saw all illness as solely having a biomedical cause and did not ask about possible social or psychological causes of pain and distress
Cultural differences	An IMG who sat back and took a history with his arms folded. This sign of respect for his culture was taken as disinterest and possible boredom by his Australian role-playing patient
Religious barriers	Intimate exams by physician of opposite gender may violate cultural or religious norms
Inappropriate examinations	An IMG who examined the liver and spleen of a patient with a nose bleed in Central Australia. He explained that this was routine in his country because of the high incidence of chronic malaria
	An IMG who examined inguinal lymph nodes on a patient who presented with back pain because, in his country, the high STI rate meant doctors would fail finals if the nodes were not checked
Diagnostic options	Either over- or underutilization of tests not readily available in their home country, such as CT scan and screening tests
Role of the doctor	An IMG who gave patients short, sharp instructions, rather than negotiating a management plan
	An IMG who always gave patients what they requested, rather than using their professional judgment to ascertain the clinical need. This included performing procedural skills beyond their expertise
Role of allied health	A doctor from East Africa struggled with the concept of health professionals being involved in post-natal depression, which he saw as a role for the grandmother and village
Therapeutic options	An IMG who only offered a script for an antibiotic and not providing analgesia, presuming that the patient would only be able to afford one medicine

their expertise can be utilized can do a lot for someone's esteem. This approach gives due respect for their skills and also demonstrates appropriate modeling for how you would like them to view your skills. It requires a different philosophical approach than occurs in the supervisory relationship with most students and residents.

Once the strengths of an IMG are known, it is time to look for the gaps. You may have sufficient information about the training, knowledge and skills of interns and residents who have been educated in your own country. When teaching IMGs, it is wise to set aside assumptions and presume you will be taking a fascinating journey into uncharted territory. Medical schools' curricula and their methods of teaching vary. For example, pathophysiology may be a gap for one learner, and another may have never been observed while conducting a physical examination. The roles of allied health providers will be novel for many, as will the epidemiology of disease. If a doctor has grown up presuming every cough is TB, it takes time to switch to think of viral upper respiratory tract infection as a likely common and benign diagnosis. As with a clinical assessment, an educational assessment consists of both subjective and objective measures.

Subjective Assessment of Skills

Small Talk in Small Towns

There is nothing like a new resident to create a buzz of excitement in small towns. As one colleague put it, "You don't see much, but what you hear makes up for it." Use your discretion to decide how much attention to pay to second- or third-hand information about the learner. Some gossip needs to be disregarded as likely to be unfair or malicious, but some may contain kernels of truth. Repeated stories of communication breakdown or unusual management may indicate issues that require attention and objective evaluation prior to a judgment and action.

Feedback from Colleagues

No doctor works in isolation and multiple health professionals "see" a resident's work in more or less overt clinical teams. Let the IMG know in advance that you will be talking to the staff and your colleagues. Document carefully any concerns expressed and then test out their veracity. Try to have a policy of only listening to such concerns if the person is prepared to write them down and is, preferably, willing to give feedback to the IMG. This approach is aimed to reduce the slow denigration of a learner and reduce the toxicity that can exist in workplaces that supposedly focus on health.

Self-identified Gaps

The IMG is likely to find gaps in their own knowledge. Ask them to keep a list either on paper or electronically. Encourage this process and take notes yourself. Unfortunately, we are not always very good at knowing what we don't know; by definition our blind spots are not visible to us and require objective assessment.

Objective Measures of Monitoring

Direct (one way mirror or "fly-on-the-wall") or indirect (audio-, videotape) observation (*see* Chapter 3) needs to be commonplace in order to gain an early sense of where the IMG learner will need the most assistance.

If you observe an unusual practice, share what you have observed and ask the IMG for their rationale for the action. Invariably, there is a good reason, but the reason may not be appropriate for their new context. From this shared space of understanding, you can both work out a possible course of action.

Actually seeing a doctor at work with patients is the best way to gauge their performance and identify blind spots. Begin by having the learner observe you first for a session or two before watching them. This gives the IMG a chance to learn from, and question, your practice before you take the role of the "fly on the wall" in their consultations. If IMGs are too shy or reticent to work with an observer or video camera, it is still possible to use audio recordings alone, with appropriate patient consent.

Colleague and Patient Feedback

Multi-source feedback is now compulsory for some residency training programs. This system requirement can provide a reasonably objective measure of how patients and colleagues perceive an IMG is performing in practice. These written notes can be compared with the norms for doctors in the same setting and can give a good basis for discussion on areas for improvement.

Assessment

Once you have collated some subjective and objective information, arrange to meet up to summarize the educational needs, and devise an initial learning plan. This can be modified over time but also can provide a useful basis for any reports you need to give to the regulatory authorities to document the IMG's educational progress. Gaps may be found across the full range of knowledge and skills expected for competent performance. It is helpful to guide the IMG about the relative importance of these gaps in their practice (*see* Table 11.2).

Consider asking the IMG to complete a learning style questionnaire so that your suggested approaches might be tailored to suit their needs. For example, if you are a "read/write" learner you may have to actively remind yourself to suggest IMG trainees consider learning from DVDs, role-playing and active experience.

Table 11.2 A Structured Approach to IMG Training

➤ Start with the doctor as a person
➤ Consider their safety and security first
➤ Ascertain their career goals
➤ Identify their learning needs and strengths
➤ Use their skills in your practice
➤ Create an educational plan
➤ Implement the plan
➤ Give regular feedback

PLAN

Implementing a learning plan is up to the IMG, with you promoting their self-reflection and providing feedback on their progress. Consider having them do more direct observation of other physicians' practices and revisit the orientation component and program goals.

Once IMGs have a few weeks of experience in a clinical setting, they may learn more about consulting and different options again from watching you or other skilled colleagues at work for a few sessions. Let them learn from watching skilled practitioners.

Local Study Group

A local study group can be a great help for IMGs preparing for exams; however, if there is no local group it is still possible to form a virtual group, and work as a team in discussing cases and doing practice exam papers or role-plays via the phone or internet. Role-plays may be unnerving and can be a very new form of learning for many IMGs. Let any IMG watch more experienced residents and IMGs practice before expecting them to join in. It is a good idea to ask the IMG to role-play as the patient prior to role-playing as the doctor in a scenario.

Problems Adapting

Some IMGs struggle to change or adapt. Although they have migrated, it can be difficult to not practice as they have always done. In some cases, there may be a firmly fixed belief that their way is the right way. If gentle persuasion and demonstration has failed to make any impact, careful confrontation may be needed. The assessment criteria from the relevant College or program standards can be cited to point out that a given treatment or attitude may be appropriate for some countries, but you would not pass an exam in this constituency. One can then help the person understand the reason for the standard, being specific about how their approach did not meet the standard, and how you can work together towards helping them reaching the standard. The possibility of failing an exam looms large, not only for professional confidence, but may also impact in terms of their immigration status. It is wise to use this concern sparingly.

Overview of Clinical Supervision

Helping IMGs adapt to work effectively in a new country is challenging but can be hugely rewarding. After an initial welcome and practical assistance, we suggest conducting a multi-faceted learning assessment and then work out a learning plan in accordance with the IMGs' career goals, learning style preference and available resources. Develop curiosity, suspend judgment and enjoy a mutual respectful learning relationship that may create lifelong friendships as well as provide quality medical care for your community.

Institutions also have a strong role to play in developing robust programs for training graduates of foreign medical programs and the next section will examine some of these challenges.

WHAT CAN INSTITUTIONS DO?

Institutions that train medical professionals are invested in finding ways to work with, and across, social and cultural differences to optimize health education, services and outcomes. Two strategies may be considered in your institution: appropriate changes to institutional climate, and faculty development. In keeping with our understanding of cultural awareness as a dynamic and relational skill, the faculty development strategies discussed in this chapter are interactive and modifiable. The institutional role is to promote the integration of cultural diversity knowledge and respect into institutional and individual policy and practice. We need to be respectful and responsive to cultural differences, while simultaneously facilitating our IMGs to navigate a new medical system and its expectations. Taking difference into account when educating IMGs can enhance the medical experiences of both the teacher and learner. This is a challenging and sometimes disorienting endeavor. Learning to work in a manner that takes difference into account in such a context is no small feat.

In 2005, Frank and MacLeod coined an institutional approach to diversity as "taking the difference into account." This approach can operate at the institutional level through policies and practices that create an *institutional climate* supportive of, and responsive to, differences, and through the effective *training of medical teachers*. It attends to the problem of "othering" those from non-dominant cultural groups by emphasizing self-awareness among teachers of IMGs.

Institutional Climate

An institution's commitment to effectively prepare teachers to meet the challenges posed by increasing diversity – cultural and other – can be measured in large part by the climate it fosters. The climate of educational institutions is an effect of many factors, including: language, policy and faculty development.

Language

Language is a primary tool of communication and, as such, plays a significant role in how attitudes towards cultural diversity are enacted and understood in medical and educational settings. The language used in teaching materials, lectures, publications and cases communicates the author's orientation to matters of difference. For example, how often are slang terms or idioms ("Hey guys," or "Run that by me") used in written or spoken language? Although these examples can seem harmless, the use of collo-quialisms can be a clue that the audience is assumed to be armed with the same cultural referents as the author, which may not be the case. In addition to cultural and ethnic differences, distinctions in class, geographic region, language and age can also make some colloquialisms unfamiliar even to multi-generational group members. Although such language is often used to encourage familiarity and to make people feel "at home," this tactic is only useful if those in the audience are already "at home" with such turns of phrase. In a diverse setting like a university or teaching hospital, this strat-egy may have the opposite effect. This is something we need to be aware of in community-based clinics with international medical postgraduate learners and patients of diverse cultures.

Policy

Creating effective policy governing educational institutions may seem like a socially or politically neutral endeavor, but policy plays a key role in taking dif-ference into account in medical education. Broadly, institutions might examine policies for ways to encourage and support critical diversity training, as well as policies that provide for the specific needs of diverse learners and teachers (such as appropriate spaces for daily prayer, or provisions for gender-specific examinations).

Faculty Development

Training Medical Teachers

Faculty development is a key strategy for institutions that train IMGs. It is important to consider the techniques used to facilitate the learning process and content. Institutions should resist the temptation to base faculty devel-opment programs for teachers of IMGs on a "deficit model" – that is, a model that constructs a culturally incompetent practitioner as one who lacks knowledge of diversity generally, or of specific facts about "diverse" groups. Instead, we should enable learners to become more aware of how culture plays a role in our own decisions, viewpoints, values, preferences, beliefs and actions, and connect this awareness to the practice of medicine and teaching. Strategies for teaching IMGs should also support teachers in prac-ticing the skills for taking difference into account as a routine part of their everyday activities.

A variety of faculty development strategies are available for teaching cultural awareness, though workshop formats or a series of short courses are generally favored in faculty development contexts. Both strategies assist with integration of new ideas into practice. Whether as a single workshop or a series of short courses, cultural awareness training is a relational learning experience and hence involves:

> reflecting on one's own cultural identity
> appreciating the diverse cultural backgrounds of IMGs
> developing communication skills that anticipate and respect cultural differences of all kinds.

The Association of Faculties of Medicine of Canada has developed a comprehensive program for both clinical supervisors and the foreign graduates and is available online (*see* resources at end of chapter).

Self-awareness: Ethnocentrism and Stereotyping

Some concepts that should be introduced early in cultural diversity training include ethnocentrism and stereotyping. Ethnocentrism, as defined by Van der Geest in 1995, refers to the belief that one's own culture is the standard against which other are judged. In the culture of medicine, ethnocentrism can be seen where clinical teachers are assumed to be "culturally neutral" whereas patients or learners may have a "culture" that must be overcome so that effective care and/or education can take place. This obscures the fact that we are all members of a culture, and we use the vantage point of our individual backgrounds to help guide our actions, thoughts and attitudes.

In 2000, Nunez defined stereotyping as the tendency to assume that all people from a cultural category will generally behave in the same ways, or hold the same beliefs. This is harmful in medical contexts because it ignores the within-group differences arising from variations in class, gender, region, age or ability, which contribute to health behaviors and disparities. Understanding ethnocentrism and stereotyping can help foster self-awareness among faculty through recognition of the ways in which our own cultural backgrounds influence our daily, professional lives.

Visual aids can help to bring the invisibility of our own culture to the forefront, stimulating the self-awareness necessary for engaging in cross-cultural education. They also appeal to visual learners and can be effective at creating or maintaining interest in new or challenging issues, such as those presented by confronting stereotypes, and social privilege.

Knowledge Transfer

Faculty development in "taking account of difference" must be applicable to the teaching context. Skills can be developed to take differences into account in teaching and professional practice. Group work is an ideal mode for developing these as it provides opportunities for faculty to practice new communication and reflective skills, and to learn from the experiences and vantage points of colleagues engaged in the same challenging process. The goal of cultural awareness training is to develop flexible and responsive communication skills for teachers of IMGs.

To that end, group exercises should offer opportunities for faculty to practice:

➤ identifying cross-cultural communication misunderstandings
➤ identifying and challenging ethnocentrism, stereotyping and discrimination
➤ exploring alternative, or less apparent, interpretations of a situation
➤ accessing resources to learn more about cultural patterns when needed
➤ using various strategies for resolving potential conflicts
➤ modeling cultural responsiveness for IMGs and helping them develop similar skills.

Teaching Skills

Just as medical students use case studies to practice their clinical skills and competencies, teachers of IMGs can use them to practice their teaching skills in context. Case studies provide scenarios relevant to the IMG-training context to which faculty can begin to apply the concepts and strategies developed through self-reflection and the practice of culturally responsive communication skills. Cases can be developed specifically for certain groups of learners, and can be modified for better application to any clinical or teaching context. The goal of case study is to enhance the skills of the faculty in identifying and responding to ethnocentrism, stereotyping, and discrimination using real life examples. They also give faculty necessary practice in applying different educational and communication strategies in teaching IMGs.

SUMMARY

Welcoming new IMGs to our education programs will take the skill and attention of the community-based clinical teacher, as well as of the institutions involved. We need to learn about them, as much as they need to know about the culture and medical system of their new home. Understanding and making explicit our own cultural assumptions is a process of self-awareness and goes hand-in-hand with learning about other cultures. These challenges overlay the medical education process in important ways. Integrating both will require creativity and patience on the part of the learner and their community-based preceptor.

FURTHER READING

Frank B, MacLeod A. Beyond the 'four Ds of multiculturalism': taking difference into account in medical education. *Med Educ.* 2005; **39**: 1178–9.
Gustafson DL, Reitmanova, S. How are we "doing" cultural diversity? A look across English Canadian undergraduate medical school programmes. *Med Teach.* 2010; **32**: 816–23.

Lockyer J, Fidler H, de Gara C, *et al.* Learning to practice in Canada: the hidden curriculum of international medical graduates. *J Contin Educ Health Prof.* 2010; **30**(1): 37–43.

MacLeod A, Frank B. Patient-centredness in a context of increasing diversity: location, location, location. *Med Teach.* 2010; **32**: 799-801.

Maslow AH. A theory of human motivation. *Psychol Rev.* 1943; **50**(4): 370–96.

Nunez, A. Transforming cultural competence into cross-cultural efficacy in women's health education. *Acad Med.* 2000; **75**: 1071–80.

Steinert Y, Walsh A, Amskel S, *et al.* *A Faculty Development Program for Teachers of International Medical Graduates.* The Association of Faculties of Medicine of Canada; 2006. Available at: www.afmc.ca/img/default_en.htm (accessed August 9, 2011).

Steinert Y, Walsh A. Introduction and program overview. In: Steinert Y, Walsh A, editors. *A Faculty Development Program for Teachers of International Medical Graduates.* Ottawa: The Association of Faculties of Medicine of Canada; 2006.

Thille P, Frank B. Educating for cultural awareness: a cultural diversity training program for teachers of internationally educated healthcare professionals. In: Steinert Y, Walsh A, editors. *A Faculty Development Program for Teachers of International Medical Graduates.* Ottawa: The Association of Faculties of Medicine of Canada; 2006.

Van der Geest, S. Overcoming ethnocentrism: how social science and medicine relate and should relate to one another. *Soc Sci Med.* 1995; **49**(7): 869–72.

VARK. *A Guide to Learning Styles.* Available at: www.vark-learn.com/english/index.asp (accessed August 9, 2011)

12

Interdisciplinary Teams

Ken Babey

Interdisciplinary collaboration in healthcare is finally finding its legs in many urban and rural environments. In rural practice, we have long explored the problem of how to perpetuate the tried and true resource of the rural generalist physician. Meanwhile, medicine has continued its path to exponentially greater complexity while successive generations of physicians have declined to commit to the long and punishing hours of work that have been the hallmark of the rural generalist physician.

It is important as community-based educators that we participate in the education process of these healthcare colleagues in constructive and appropriate ways. It is equally important that we understand the potential scope and limitations of each discipline, as we share our experience with them. In the past, what we thought of as interdisciplinary in community practice was the addition of a Nurse Practitioner (NP) to our practice and, then, a loose assemblage of other community resources, such as dieticians, community mental health workers and diabetic educators. Where these disciplines have been embraced and the professionals practicing them are appropriately prepared, trained and funded, the collaborative benefit can be substantial. Much effort has been expended to expose medical students (and those from other health disciplines) to this concept of Interdisciplinary Healthcare (IDHC). With the proliferation of courses, publications and field experience in the subject, it must be the rare student who remains unexposed.

Traditionally, professionals nurtured their own kind, with physicians teaching medical students and postgraduate physicians, nurses teaching nurses and teachers teaching teachers. There is now opportunity and growing community obligation to share knowledge across disciplines in the endeavors of teaching, learning and day-to-day-work. There are good models for this concept in many Academic Health Science Centers, but a lack of them in community-based practices (*see* Table 12.1).

Concurrent with the trend to distributed education of health professionals, many regions have also seen increased opportunities for the development of

Interdisciplinary Health Teams (IDHTs). The somewhat parallel development of these trends has presented some opportunities and challenges. Here we focus on one of those: how to teach in an IDHT. Within this developing matrix of care and health education there are at least four different kinds of teaching.

Table 12.1 Types of Interdisciplinary Teaching and Learning

➤ *Homogenous:* Teaching students of the same discipline the concept and workings of the IDHT, e.g. doctors teaching medical students within the IDHT

➤ *Heterogonous:* Teaching students of a different discipline an appropriate subset of skills and the meshing of the team as a whole, e.g. physician teaching Nurse Practitioner or Physician Assistant shared skills and how to function in the team

➤ *Disseminated:* The teaching of existing health team members the value of integration with their colleagues, usually by exposing them to students or practitioners of a "new" discipline, e.g. introducing the Physician Assistant to physician colleagues through mentorship

➤ *Reciprocal:* Bidirectional learning when new disciplines are integrated into the team, e.g. the physician learning effective collaboration with the clinical Pharmacist and vice versa.

HOW IS INTERDISCIPLINARY TEACHING SIMILAR?

Most aspects of good teaching practice apply across all professions. What is always needed is space and time. What is increasingly needed for the clinical teacher to stay in the game is the ability to change and adapt. Intergenerational differences are more pronounced than in the past, with the proliferation of learning technologies. Adopting an online and linked-in culture is not essential but it will be the culture of all students. "You Tube" becomes a preferred teacher and memory is served with "Apps" on an ever-present hand-held device. Within this setting, the clinician teacher must temper Practice Guidelines with experiential decision-making or evidence-informed practice. Fortunately, most teaching programs provide regular faculty development workshops where problem-solving (regarding the student–teacher relationship) and teaching theory are reviewed.

Providing a Fertile Learning Environment in the IDHT

To provide a fertile learning environment in the community setting it is important that the interdisciplinary team be supported by good leadership. Without it, the promise of the rich inter-relationships in an IDHT is diminished and the dynamics can be poisoned. This is readily observed by the learner and makes for a poor interdisciplinary collaboration experience. For example, an NP is brought into a physician group to provide urgent care within her scope of practice; the physicians all have different expectations, some beyond her scope and some menial and not approaching the limits of her scope. With no leadership to address the issue, both the NP and physicians are unhappy and an attending student has a diminished view of the synergy.

A well-developed system of communication between the disciplines that is understood by all is essential if the student is to enjoy the full benefit of the multidisciplinary collaboration. An effort should be made to invite the whole team to participate in the education process when a learner is aboard. If all professionals do not feel part of the process they function only as a button to be pushed rather than a teaching resource.

The experience of multidisciplinary rounds or a case conference is perhaps an illustration of the team at its best. Although they can be time-consuming, they can, with experience and leadership, be brief and productive. These are often held out by students to be the best illustrations of the "real-life Problem-Based Learning" (PBL) and offer an excellent opportunity to see who the players are.

In its simplest form, the field experience for students in the health disciplines is mentorship. Whether we have a Physician–Physician Assistant (PA) or a Physician–NP mentorship the tendency is some form of "see one – do one – teach one" (observation, imitation and reinforcement). That is, we observe while we let the learner safely determine their skill/confidence quotient. We then give them more or less freedom to do what we do with variable degrees of observation and feedback. Ideally, we do this in an adaptive or contextual way, making our support and direction proportional to their confidence and competence. The concept of learning by doing is, in many ways, why students seek community field placements. These same communities often lack the high-tech models for simulation. What they offer is practical education.

It is this practical education that leads to the "Ah Ha moments" that are best retained and foster the development of confidence.

HOW IS INTERDISCIPLINARY TEACHING DIFFERENT?

The students from different disciplines (e.g. pharmacy, medicine and NP) have vastly different educational backgrounds. Each discipline has its own culture and its own scope of practice with which the preceptor should be conversant. They may even have different concepts of ethics.

Different disciplines are often ignorant of each other's fields and how they approach the same problem (e.g. the Chiropractor and Physician may see a sore back differently and interpret the same X-rays very differently, but offer very complementary care to a patient). Students will often be found to have crossed disciplines in their training. Consider the experienced obstetrical nurse training as an NP or an experienced military combat medic as a PA. Many of these are seeking a broader scope of professional practice and greater level of challenge in their careers.

Because these students are seeking to expand their role with less time in "higher education" than the medical students whose process is more familiar to the teacher, it behooves the preceptor to entertain the questions: "Do they have enough knowledge to back up their action?" "Do they know what they don't know?" "Are they too adventurous and are they risk-takers?" These are not necessarily considered negative qualities, but need to be evaluated in the context of patent safety and best practice.

Patient expectations may be at variance with the skills or limitations of the learner. In distributed education settings, the patients will not usually have had exposure to a NP or PA until you have one in your office as a student. The patient may be moderately tolerant of a medical student, but less so of a student clinician whose role they do not understand. It pays to post a statement in office and waiting room about the role of interdisciplinary learners and to introduce the idea in local press and other public media. Having one or two of the more excellent students for a rotation will reassure your patients as to their value as clinicians.

MAKING IT WORK
Leadership and Relationships

It takes time and sometimes a champion to break down barriers while creating and expanding an IDHT. Introducing a PA student, for example, into an IDHT and/or a hospital setting when none of the team has experienced the PA before can be time-consuming and loaded with misunderstandings and roadblocks. Careful preparation of the staff about roles, relationships and limitations where they exist are important. Fortunately, a single student who is a good salesperson and role model for their discipline can break down most interprofessional barriers. The introduction of students of that profession who follow, find less resistance and more acceptance.

Likewise, bringing a newly trained professional into the team can require the same cautions plus some active teaching of the existing staff. An example would be bringing a Pharmacist into an IDHT. The pharmacist may know his business and proceed to mine the practice files for poly-pharmacy and dangerous drug interactions as well as best practices (as in "not being met") and proceed to supply long missives to the physicians on how they might change their practice. This approach will certainly alienate the physician core. A good physician/champion/mentor will help the pharmacist to learn to be brief and constructive. The adapted pharmacist can now mesh effectively with clinicians/physicians and find ways to expand their teaching skills to benefit the team, such as with smoking cessation counseling and asthma education.

Professional Cultures

Crossing cultures can be tricky in interdisciplinary teaching. A good example is in the Medicine–NP interface. The scope of practice for an NP is well-defined by their regulatory body. The educational process might be the sharing of a certain subset of skills between physician and NP. Is this subset best taught by the physician who can demonstrate how theory is modified by practice? Does familiarity with the whole set foster better understanding of the subset of knowledge required? Unfortunately, because of the cultural chasm between the medical and nursing professions, physicians often do not have the opportunity to participate in the training of NPs. When the opportunity arises, it can provide a rewarding experience and insight for both physician-mentor and NP student, as well as providing a level of comfort for both participants in future collaborative practice. An interesting further issue regarding culture is the potential lack of acceptance by other nursing staff of the nurse who leaves that discipline to receive NP training then returns to the same workplace in a new capacity.

Teaching Techniques

It is interesting that students of all disciplines who reach community-based education placements tend to be motivated to independence and attracted to the greater opportunity for hands-on experience than they can often receive at an urban tertiary care center. When we multiply this quality by the number of types of health professions that we may be called upon to teach, and their varied backgrounds, the idea of an Adaptive Mentorship is worth considering in detail. A good preceptor knows when to teach and when to observe or listen. Learners often come to us with an excellent knowledge base. More facts are often not what are needed. The experienced clinical teacher exposes his or her knowledge bank helpfully, as a living PBL exercise. She can share a tolerance for variance that allows the learner to apply their knowledge and understanding to decision-making in a practical way, not just by application of rigid practice guidelines without having to think.

Sharing "war stories" of challenging past experiences that illustrate a point or problem-solving process is a favorite learning tool for students of all disciplines. It allows the learner access to the teacher as a person and provides ready-made experience that is easily remembered.

In the IDHT, it quickly becomes apparent to the student (often more than to the teacher) that different people and different disciplines do certain things well. Within a team setting, it is worthwhile to encourage the student to learn from these specific talents. It is easy for students of all health disciplines to fall into the pattern of linear thinking. When teaching in multiple disciplines where knowledge may run to various depths, it seems rewarding to emphasize lateral thinking to broaden and enrich each discussion, away from simple pattern recognition. It is stimulating and valuable for learners and clinicians alike to learn and share the recognition of "red flags." It is a tribute to the team and a benefit to the patient when the dietician recognizes and reports increasing depression or the NP recognizes the sore shoulder as polymyalgia.

When the "pre-dedicated" learner arrives at a community field placement ("I just want to do neuro-ophthalmology"), do not give up on them. Their experience in a multidisciplinary setting may still influence their career choice, or at least help them to be more understanding consultants when they receive a consult request from the NP or PA.

SUMMARY

Interdisciplinary teaching brings new and likely unfamiliar challenges to community-based practices. Each practice and community will have to determine what their health professional needs are. In order to maintain and enhance services, community-based preceptors may decide to invest their energy in interdisciplinary teaching. Because it moves us outside the "box," leadership and clarity of roles and expectations are important elements if true healthcare "teams" are going to develop. As various models develop, it will be informative to see which ones are best suited to community-based environments.

FURTHER READING

Bradshaw MJ, Lowenstein AJ. *Innovative Teaching Strategies in Nursing & Related Health Professions*. 5th ed. MA: Jones & Bartlett Publishers; 2010.

Canadian Interprofessional Health Collaborative. Available at: www.cihc.ca

Collier R. Verdict still out on family health teams. *CMAJ*. 2011; **183**(10): 1131–2.

Dienst E, Byl N. Evaluation of an education program in healthcare teams. *J Comm Health*. 1981; **6**(4): 282–98.

Firth J. Levels and sources of stress in medical students. *BMJ*. 1986; **292**: 1177–80.

Interprofessional Rural Program of B.C. (IRPbc). Available at: www.irpbc.com

Kolb D. *Experiential Learning: experience as the source of learning and development*. Columbus, OH: Prentice Hall; 1983.

Ralph E, Walker K. *Rising with the Tide: Applying Adaptive Mentorship in the Professional Practicum*. *Collected Essays of Learning and Teaching (CELT)*, Vol 3. Hamilton ON: Society for Teaching and Learning in Higher Education (STLHE), from a workshop presented for STLHE Fredericton NB; June 2009.

Rodriguez-Paz J. Beyond see one, do one, teach one: toward a different training paradigm. *Qual Saf Healthcare*. 2009; **1**: 63–8.

Vozenilek J. See one, do one, teach one, advanced technology in medical education. *Acad Emerg Med*. 2004; **11**(11): 1496–1502.

Zuckerman M. Dimensions of sensation seeking. *J Consul Clin Psychol*. 1971; **36**(1): 45–52.

Zuckerman, M. (1990) The psychophysiology of sensation seeking. *Journal of Personality*. 1990; **8**(1): 313–345.

Zull, J. The art of changing the brain. *Educ Leadership*. 2004; **62**(1): 68–72.

13

Inner City Rotations

Michael Dillon and Sasha Ho Ferris Nyriabu

When many medical students imagine a family doctor, the picture of a small-town GP may spring to mind, perhaps with home visits after office hours to attend to the elderly or infirm, or to assess an ill child. In recent decades, however, the picture of the family doctor has changed along with the demographics of our communities. In North America, our populations have been progressively increasing in urban and suburban areas, while declining in rural communities. While the majority of care providers in North America practice in urban centers, most family practices will be populated by those patients who have the wherewithal to find a doctor and maintain a relationship in "typical" office practices. The city core, however, is home to a large underserviced population living on society's margins. These patients typically experience great difficulty gaining access to and maintaining primary healthcare in family practices. It is not distance that separates this community from the mainstream, but differences. Many of these differences are reflected in the social determinants of health, such as poverty, safety and housing.

To respond to these challenges, medical practices serving people in such settings must adapt the "book learning" of medical school to the realities of inner city healthcare delivery. While many physicians are able to support solo or small group practices, inner city medicine is increasingly practiced in multi-professional clinics. Such clinics will often utilize teams of professionals involved in collaborative care, with different avenues for patients to gain access to the healthcare system, and innovative modes for care delivery that respect the socio-economic underpinnings of illness and healing. It is essential for "inner city" healthcare providers and their students to appreciate the importance of recognizing the social determinants of health in their practices.

UNIQUENESS OF INNER CITY MEDICINE
What is it that differentiates inner city practices from other general practice settings?

Urban medical teaching often begins in the somewhat cloistered worlds of tertiary care hospitals and academic teaching centers. While many such institutions are by definition situated in larger urban centers, there are often barriers to developing relationships with certain clientele, particularly those who are homeless or under-housed, or whose lifestyles or mental health conditions pose barriers to the manner in which they gain access to healthcare. These patients can be seen as constituting a community by virtue of where they live and who they are: minorities, refugees and mental health patients living in poverty.

Inner city practices will often make efforts to lower barriers, and provide ways of allowing a diverse range of clientele to gain access to on-going healthcare. While community-based preceptors who work in such practices need no reminding of the challenges faced by provider and patient alike, they need to be able to impart to their students, not only knowledge of the important medical issues faced by their inner city clientele, but also sensitivity to the range of social and economic factors many people face in the core areas of our cities. It is important for the community-based teacher to integrate a learner's required curriculum with care provision that is sensitive to the needs of a diverse clientele.

Additionally, there are particular health concerns that predominate in inner city medical practices, including HIV, hepatitis, tuberculosis, addiction and mental health issues. Patients who are poor and socially marginalized have worse health and die earlier than people in more stable situations. Care delivery in inner city practices must address the larger societal issues while simultaneously providing care for individuals and families.

EDUCATIONAL CONTENT AND CONTEXT

Since this is a challenging clinical environment, not surprisingly, teaching and learning take on new context and content. Establishing a safe learning environment needs to ensure the learner is not overwhelmed emotionally or cognitively. This will include close supervision and access to their preceptor and a graded exposure and delegation of responsibility to this complex clinical setting. As we shall see, any single case can itself become overwhelming and require multi-faceted considerations and interventions. An orientation to the practice team and how to access them is also an important part of getting started.

The content of the medical presentations will often have a concentration of substance abuse, psychiatric and infectious disease not typically seen by the learner outside of specialty clinics. The context of the patient–doctor interaction will also be novel for most learners. Patients may not have living quarters and access to clean clothes. They may be afraid to visit a pharmacy or see a new member of the treatment team. There are safety issues for the learner, preceptor, staff and patient: from attention to universal precautions to the safe management of weapons. Such clinical environments will have developed implicit and explicit practices and the learner will need to be oriented appropriately.

The educational objective of inner city rotations is to allow the learner to understand the clientele and the problems they deal with in a comprehensive, compassionate and continuous manner. Exposure to, and understanding of, inner city medicine will inevitably help to ensure recruitment of future care providers into such practices, and so ensure the on-going sustainability of the care-provider pool in these communities. In the following series of fictionalized cases, we will outline key elements of teaching and essential attributes of the learner.

CASE SCENARIOS

In these cases, the social determinants of health will be recognized, and the cases will illustrate teaching points that help to develop the Medical Learner as:
➤ Health Advocate
➤ Professional
➤ Expert Clinician
➤ Communicator
➤ Collaborator
➤ Culturally Competent Clinician
➤ Scholar

"Robbie": a Challenging Client

Robbie is 45 years old. He is a new patient who has recently been accepted into on-going care at your clinic after being discharged from hospital on treatment for active tuberculosis. He has been dealing with issues of chronic pain and substance use. He has a past history of incarceration. Robbie has walked in requesting to be seen today to get help with problems of an increase in his chronic pain due to having been recently assaulted in his apartment. Additionally, he has been having difficulties with side-effects of his TB medications.

Robbie is to be seen by a medical student on her first clinical rotation. How can you help her triage today's problems and develop a mutually satisfactory plan of action?

Often people who live in core areas of cities will have dealt with issues related to poverty, violence and abuse. In order to survive the "mean streets" many, of necessity, develop ways of interaction that may seem "hard" or "rough." The preceptor's comfort with the clientele and the problems faced can do much to set the learner at ease, and to provide the patient with a supportive clinical environment in which to receive a fair health assessment. In dealing with such clientele, the preceptor will need to guide the learner to develop the following traits.

The Learner as Communicator

This includes a non-judgemental attitude in conversation and history taking and respect for the mutual safety of the patient, student and healthcare providers. We need to understand the patient's agenda for the visit and reconcile this with issues brought forward by the healthcare provider and the learner.

In this scenario, the learner will begin by asking the patient what he is hoping from today's visit. As it turns out, Robbie is requesting a narcotic pain reliever as he has been buying narcotics "on the street" to help cope with the pain. He is also complaining of loss of appetite related to his anti-TB therapy.

The clinician's agenda includes a review of the "safety" of today's visit, and may involve asking about any pertinent or active legal charges either placed by or against the patient.

Furthermore, it may be advisable to ask about any weapons the patient may have brought into the office, and offer to "check" them in a secure place while care is being delivered. Importantly, the clinical agenda must involve strategies to help Robbie finish his TB treatment.

The Learner as Collaborator

The learner may be directed to try to help Robbie deal with today's symptoms in a medically safe and compassionate manner. If narcotic pain reliever or other medications of possible abuse are to be prescribed, careful review of the patient's request must be done with the supervising clinician. Using regional or national guidelines may help guide clinical decision-making in the prescription of narcotics for non-malignant pain. Using the "harm-reduction" principle, the controlled provision of certain medications, under specific circumstances, may help to divert the patient from using "street drugs" and the many associated potential harms while important health issues are addressed. For Robbie, the provision of anti-nausea medications and a referral to the team's dietician may help with his nausea and his nutritional status. An analgesic prescription, perhaps with a "narcotic use contract" may be negotiated.

Finally, to help the patient finish his TB treatment, you may guide your learner to help Robbie understand the benefits for himself and the community of successfully eradicating his infection. However, Robbie may need further "buy-in." Many publicly run TB programs will actually provide small "rewards" for successful completion of treatment. In Robbie's case, he informs the medical student that his is fond of the music of Captain Beefheart and The Magic Band. As it happens, the student is able to procure a copy of "Trout Mask Replica" from the neighborhood CD shop, and Robbie is promised the CD upon completion of the TB therapy, by which time his pain has settled, requiring only simple non-prescription analgesia.

"Janis": a Sex Trade Worker/Vulnerable Woman

"Janis" is a 25-year-old Aboriginal woman presenting to be seen for severe pain in her throat. She is known to be involved in sex work and is a frequent cocaine user. She also has evidence of learning disabilities related to Fetal Alcohol Spectrum Disorder, and is known to have an extremely chaotic living situation. Your learner is a PA student early in training. How can you direct the learner to best help Janis?

The Learner as Professional

Guide the student to develop an attitude of "open curiosity." One does not need to know everything, but how to ask. Do not try to be "too cool." Try to avoid language with the patient that is too "technical" and when needed use "common translations" of medical terminology, but do maintain professional demeanor. Ensure that the patient is as comfortable as possible during the interview.

The Learner as Communicator

After establishing comfort and rapport with the patient, the learner must then obtain a sexual history. The learner is instructed to remember that sex work is an occupation that is a "necessary evil" for many, and carries with it high occupational hazards. The learner should be given direction to obtain a thorough sexual history from this patient (as with any patient with concerns potentially related to sexual health). The learner should inquire about recent sexual contacts, types of sexual practices, physical assault or forced sex.

Similarly, this is an opportunity to ask about substance use. The majority of sex workers will have some degree of trouble involving drugs and addictions. While the education of healthcare professionals will usually address some of the aspects of substance use and addiction (the "who" and the "why," for example), the training of most health professionals does not usually include the specifics of "how." The care-provider trainee will, therefore, learn important information from the patient by asking him or her to describe the details of their technique of substance use, as these may be important clues to sorting out a patient's presenting concerns as well as decreasing transmission for blood-borne illness. In this instance, the PA student should determine: the particulars of Janis' substance use, what drug (clarify if unfamiliar street names or terminology is used), what route (smoked, sniffed or snorted, swallowed, injected), with whom (sharing needles, crack pipes, possible cross-contamination of common equipment such as spoons, water, filters, other paraphernalia associated with drug use).

The Learner as Expert Clinician

The learner is directed to perform a careful examination, with the patient's permission. In circumstances such as this, the presence of a "chaperone," such as a nurse (preferably of the same gender as the patient) is advisable, not only for medico-legal purposes but also for support for the patient.

Inspection of the oral cavity would include inspection for ulcers, trauma, or other breaks in the mucosa. Inflammation of the posterior pharynx and tonsillar area may indicate inflammation or exudate. Similarly, examination of the genitals and anus may be important, particularly if there were a history of unprotected sexual contact, or symptoms of pain, discomfort or discharge.

In Janis's case, her symptoms suggest pharyngitis. As such, a swab for streptococcus and/or rapid strep test would be helpful. Additionally, testing the oropharynx for chlamydia and gonorrhea should be performed. It is important to remind the learner that the nucleic acid amplification test kits for cervical or urethral chlamydial and gonorrheal infections cannot be used for testing of other sites, such as the oral cavity, conjunctiva or rectum. Testing of these sites must be done using swabs for culture swabs for gonorrhea and viral cultures for visible lesions. Supplemental serology should always be obtained (with patient consent) for sexually transmissible or blood–borne conditions such as HIV, hepatitis B and C and syphilis. Viral illnesses such as hepatitis C have been shown to be transmissible by sharing crack cocaine pipes.

The student should identify whether there has been some establishment of trust and rapport with the patient. The history should be summarized and a set of differential diagnoses proposed. The differential postulated for her sore throat could include: strep throat; viral pharyngitis; mononucleosis; gonorrheal, chlamydial pharyngitis or local irritant effects of drugs.

With supplemental history taking, Janis reveals that there was an "equipment malfunction" with her crack pipe, and a small metallic mesh screen which was part of the pipe came loose on inhalation, and the hot piece of metal had been inhaled into the oropharynx where it lodged, creating a local burn. The patient was able to pull the screen out, leaving behind a small burnt area of mucosa. The plan would be to treat the patient symptomatically and leave the lesion to heal spontaneously. Treatment with antibiotics was offered on spec in advance of test results due to additional risk factors for STI exposure via unprotected oral sex with a male client.

The Learner as Health Advocate

Your student could be directed to review issues related to the safety of Janis' work and living situations, and offer assistance as indicated, e.g. ensuring that the patient has an adequate supply of condoms, and offer a return visit for test results and possibly further testing after the "window period" of false seronegativity has passed for HIV, hepatitis and syphilis. It is an unfortunate reality that minority women are more likely than the norm to have been affected by violence, sexual abuse and assault. This, in combination with injection drug use, puts these women at particularly high risk of contraction of HIV infection, as well as hepatitis B, C and syphilis. In the case of a patient such as Janis, engagement in supportive programming that is respectful of culture and traditions may lead along the path to recovery.

Exploring options for safer housing and financial supports can be steps in the right direction to help Janis off the streets. The involvement of a Social Worker may lead Janis to connections with specialty services aimed at helping those involved in sex work or to support services for those affected by FASD. Small steps and "one suggestion at a time" may be the best strategies to achieving on-going rapport and eventual change in life situation for patients like Janis.

"The Katanga Family": the Refugee Family

There are eight people crammed into your largest examination room. They are the Katangas, a Congolese family that has just arrived from Kenya where they have been living in a United Nations Refugee Camp for the past five years. You are working with a second year Family Medicine Resident who has just started her elective at your clinic. In anticipation of the interview with this family, how do you prepare your Resident to meet the Katanga family?

The Learner as a Culturally Competent Clinician

When faced with the unknown and unexpected, even experienced clinicians may feel daunted or anxious. When dealing with the healthcare of newcomers, the challenges are manifold. To help the learner before the clinical interaction with a newcomer family, the following issues must be considered: communication, geographical and environmental concerns, intra-family dynamics, medical concerns, including mental health and trauma history. With these concerns in mind, you may instruct your Family Medicine Resident in the following skills.

Communication

Anyone who has traveled for business or pleasure to a country where the language differs from one's own can appreciate the stresses posed by the difficulties in understanding and being understood. In this case, it is crucial to plan in advance, whenever possible, to have trained, professional language interpreters available for the clinical interview. It is generally preferable to have "in-person" interpreter services whenever possible, as this generally helps improve the patients' comfort, and allows for the interpretation of body language and emotion. Increasingly, however, there are excellent interpreter services available by telephone, and these should be used when an in-person interpreter service is not available. The use of other family members or friends as interpreters should be avoided, as the potential for misinterpretation and misunderstanding is high. In particular, the use of children as interpreters is particularly troublesome.

Geographical and Environmental Concerns

Let us imagine, for example, that you are a clinician in cold climate. The Katanga family whom you are about to assess has just recently arrived. Last week they were in Kenya and it was 38°C (100°F) in the daytime. They have never experienced temperatures below freezing, let alone a landscape covered in ice and snow. Addressing these obvious, but often unstated concerns, may help to increase patients' comfort and allow for a more satisfactory subsequent assessment. An age-old conversation starter, discussing the weather can take on practical and social importance.

Initial Assessment

In the case of the Katanga Family, the initial visit may be an opportunity to introduce them to the local health system, provide advice on how to get help in the case of medical concerns or emergencies. The learner may also obtain a collective history, as generally families of newcomers have similar if not identical migration histories, and were often living in the same physical settings prior to departure for their new homes. This is also an opportunity to develop a genogram for the family, which can be copied and put into individual family members' medical files.

Medical Concerns

Many clinicians will feel uncomfortable when faced with medical scenarios which are unexpected or infrequently encountered. In the case of newcomer refugees, these anxieties may be amplified by concerns related the tropical, parasitic or other "exotic" health concerns relatively rare in "developed" or "western" countries. Furthermore, the prevalence of mental health concerns and post-traumatic stress disorder may be quite significant, depending on the experiences prior to migration: torture, violence, rape and sexual abuse, witnessed murder or forced homicide. Often, such concerns are left "buried," but the clinician and trainee must be vigilant to recognize significant mental health concerns and be prepared to offer appropriate supports as necessary.

The Medical Learner as Scholar

In the case of this family, the Family Medicine Resident may be directed to finish the initial history, and arrange for a follow-up visit with the family. In the interim, the learner may explore local community resources to assist with subsequent assessment. This may prove a valuable opportunity to advance the supervising clinician's own knowledge base. Reading around these patients could include tropical disease, recent socio-political events, post-traumatic stress disorder, to name a few. Having a world atlas may become a useful office text. Using such information, the learner may develop his or her knowledge base, provide a higher level of care for the patients, and contribute to the on-going growth of the teacher's own clinical practice.

CONCLUSION

A highly functioning inner city teaching practice will encourage the learner to be knowledgeable and competent, skilled in communication, reflection and conflict resolution, and affirmative to patients and colleagues alike, engendering attitudes of mutual respect, trust and a spirit of collaboration. The learner will be guided down the pathway of "lifelong learning" while appreciating the role of healthcare provider as "advocate," aware that understanding the socio-economic determinants of health is as important as diagnoses and treatments themselves.

Learning and working in an inner city community clinic fosters a deeper appreciation for the diversity of cultures, social issues and difficulties of access that are key elements in inner city healthcare. The training received in such inner-city settings will enhance subsequent capacity to practice and serve in a diversity of settings, whether in remote and rural communities or a city clinic by a busy transit line.

Finally, the learner will develop perspective on the local, regional and national healthcare systems, will understand that every system has finite resources and, as such, it is an individual and collective responsibility to work continuously toward more cost-effective models of care to increase access to healthcare for to all, particularly those most in need.

FURTHER READING

Wasylenki D. Inner city health. *CMAJ*. 2001; **164**(2): 215.

Fernandez L, MacKinnon S, Silver J, editors. Spatially-concentrated racialized poverty as a social determinant of health: the case of Winnipeg's inner city. In: *The Social Determinants of Health in Manitoba, Canadian Centre for Policy Alternatives*. Winnipeg, Manitoba: Institute of Child Health; 2010; pp. 161–3.

Walker P, Barnett E, editors. *Immigrant Medicine*. Saunders Elsevier; 2007.

Pottie K, Tugwell P, Feightner J, *et al.* on behalf of the Canadian Collaboration for Immigrant and Refugee Health (CCIRH). Evidence-based clinical guidelines for immigrants and refugees. *CAMJ* 2011; **183**(12): E824–925. DOI: 10.1503/camj.090313.

Websites

www.uwinnipeg.ca/index/cms-filesystem-action?file=pdfs/factsheets/factsheet-urban-
and-inner-city-studies.pdf

www.stmichaelshospital.com/research/crichprofilelist.php

nationalpaincentre.mcmaster.ca/opioid

14

Rural Rotations

Len Kelly

INTRODUCTION

Rural medical experiences present some challenges and many benefits to the learner, preceptor, community and universities involved. There are intrinsic and extrinsic rewards for all of those involved. The intrinsic benefits are subtle but real, and speak to quality of social and professional life: social capital, enjoyment and enthusiasm. The extrinsic advantages are bankable: recruitment of the next generation of physicians, and economic development, for example.

We know that facilitating rural applicants to medical schools is the first ingredient for achieving a sustainable rural workforce. Many medical schools are now recognizing their social accountability responsibilities toward under-serviced areas and populations and are encouraging and facilitating more rural students to apply. This often requires creative community outreach and application assistance. If these efforts are successful in a professional generation, we will likely see an increasing number of physicians who themselves grew up in rural areas. The second internationally accepted ingredient for recruiting future rural physicians is providing medical education opportunities in these rural and remote areas. What effect do these have?

UNDERGRADUATE TRAINING

Some medical programs have developed a year-long rural clinical clerkship. In 2008, Worley looked at students who were 5–7 years on from the third year of medical studies in Australia. He found that, even controlling for student's rural background, rurally placed clerks were 19 times more likely to now be in a rural practice setting. This study stands alongside many others that connect the dots between rural educational placements and successful careers in rural practice. More distributed learning initiatives are being established in rural areas with excellent academic and clinical results. In the new Northern Ontario School of Medicine in Canada, the recently graduated charter class chose family medicine residencies at a rate double that of the national average. This may be a result of their eight-month clinical clerkship in a rural setting which demonstrates to the students the broad scope and satisfaction of a rural career as a generalist.

An American rural medical student recruiting and admission program in Illinois, which began in 1993, has seen 64% of its graduates end up in primary care practices in rural areas. One of the oldest American rural undergraduate initiatives, WWAMI (Wyoming, Washington, Alaska, Montana and Idaho) has been integrating student selection and undergraduate medical education for over 30 years. They achieve over 60% of their graduates in primary care and 23% in rural practices – double that of their peers in traditional programs.

A fully distributed four-year medical program is the next step, currently being taken in the remote Northern Territories of Australia by Flinders University. It will be very informative to follow the outcomes of such fully rural medical educational initiatives.

Lesser exposure is more common and still has effective recruitment potential. Four- to eight-week rural rotations at Monash University demonstrated that students from an urban background were four times more likely to consider a rural career after even such a short rotation. Students who grew up in a rural area and had some rural undergraduate experience were nine times more predisposed. These findings highlight the two commonly accepted predictors of rural practice: rural background and rural educational placements. The evidence to this point is that the more, the better. Strasser's Monash study pointed out the next link in the chain: postgraduate rural placements.

POSTGRADUATE TRAINING

Internship and residency programs need to offer adequate rural experiences if they are to build on the students' undergraduate exposure. For many schools, that is the next step: primary care and specialty mandatory rotations. That way there is a visible and consistent rural pathway available to those who choose it and a clear commitment to remote and underserved communities. Only one of the rural postgraduate models in the USA includes a small number of residents involved in continuous rural three-year family medicine programs. The approach of the other 13 schools with a rural training track is the "one – two" model, with the first year's training in an urban hospital and the remaining two in a rural location. The results have been promising, with 76% of residents ending up in rural practice, but there have only been a total of 107 graduates to this point.

Australian rural postgraduate training can be achieved through two colleges. Each takes 4 years for a rural fellowship with between 1 and 3 years in rural settings. The creation of these competing schemes is recent and outcomes measures are not yet available.

The Canadian standard for a rural family medicine residency program designation is six months of the total 24 months of training. Currently 20% of family medicine positions are designated rural, but no national estimates of subsequent rural practice location are known. Clearly different international medical education constituencies struggle with postgraduate rural training and its overall integration with even successful undergraduate programs. This is the next hurdle for completing the continuous chain of rural training.

Not all students are bound for a rural generalist career. There is benefit for even the urban-based specialist physician to have been exposed to rural communities and their medical capacity during their training. These specialists will better understand the difficulty their rural patients encounter when they travel great distances for appointments. They may appropriately minimize the number of required follow-up visits, or be more willing to participate in more videoconferencing for follow-up discussions. They will also understand the capabilities and limitations of their rural physician colleagues. Rural exposure can only facilitate better communication and case management and shared follow-up for rural patients.

As in all primary care experiences, the learner encounters undifferentiated patient presentations. Urban teaching hospital rotations sample the tip of the "patient pyramid" where those admitted are a selected subset of the total. Less differentiated and diagnosed patients will be looked after locally and as outpatients. They may have documented symptoms without the arrival of a diagnosis, sometimes with resolution and no treatment. It is good for learners to see the larger part of the pyramid where symptoms prevail and uncertainty keeps them company.

CORE vs ELECTIVE ROTATIONS

Just as learners at different educational levels are given graded patient responsibility, the same applies to their teachers. Initially, in our teaching careers, we may be exposed to elective students and residents and we may develop a particular style of teaching. However, when we become involved with supervising prolonged rotations of several months, we are assuming greater educational responsibility. We can cut fewer corners: the educational "buck" has stopped here. Our feedback and evaluations are central to the learners' education and progression in their program. Our input is no longer tangential to that of another, more informed assessment. The relationship and role are qualitatively as well as quantitatively different. A four-month rotation is not merely four times longer that a one-month one. It means that a significant proportion of learning, supervising and monitoring are expected (and need) to occur.

So, when a preceptor takes on this more significant educational role, the rotation they supervise has moved from an elective to a core rotation. The rotation now assumes a central position in the student's learning. We need to maintain many of our positive attributes but also need to "change gears" as we might in cycling up a longer hill if we wish to maintain the same teaching and learning pace. Core rotations call upon us to ensure that learning objectives are met, that a broad scope of patient care has been offered to the learner, and that we have delved deeper into their learning potential. It may require us to invest more time and energy into our teaching role. We may notice shortcomings in our teaching skills that may need support from fellow clinical teachers or focused faculty development. These core rotations not only raise the educational bar for community-based medical educators but also for the learners.

LEARNER'S EXPERIENCE

Students in rural rotations work closely with their clinical teachers. These physicians can facilitate some unique lessons. A 2004 Australian study of medical students by Worley and colleagues found that community-based students had a richer experience than their urban hospital-based colleagues. They reported greater patient contact and increased time supervised by an experienced clinician. Rural rotations are rich educational opportunities for personal growth, in addition to being high-quality educational experiences (*see* Figure 14.1).

There is no anonymity for either the student or their preceptor in a small community. This brings more familiarity to any patient–doctor interaction. This may be a novel experience for the learner, who may have only encountered

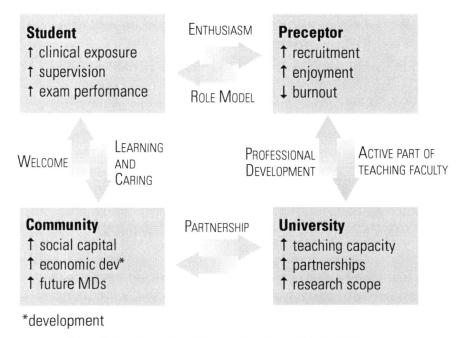

Figure 14.1 Theoretical Model of Distributed Medical Education

unknown patients in urban hospitals to this point in their short career. Discussions about relationships and boundaries become common topics.

Living in a small community for one month or one year gives a reciprocal shared look at one another for both the learner and the population.

"Would I like to work and live in a place similar to this?"
"Would my partner, family thrive here?"
"Would this professional "fit in" if they came back to practice here?"
"Will they return after their training is completed?"
"Would I want them as my family doctor?"

It is hard to predict the development of career interests, attitudes and the relationships that can occur. Even a trained physician moving to a small community needs to "try it on" to see if they and the community are a good fit for one another. Schooling for the physician's children and spousal contentment are key reasons in the literature of the "departing" rural physician, and these will be major issues in choosing a practice community. Students these days seem very hesitant to commit to a particular practice once they graduate. In primary care they seem to fear the perceived role of the overworked generalist locked into a difficult lifestyle. We need to share with our learners the joys of small community life, as well as its limitations – that it is not all work!

ROLE IN THE COMMUNITY

When a student is accepted into your community for training, they become a part of your professional group. One may need to share with them that their public activities will always be noticed. They need to exhibit respectful behavior even outside work. If they have a longer rotation and are able to know patients more, they should be prepared for patients asking personal medical questions on the street or even in the grocery store! They will need to have a benign phrase prepared to deflect the public discussion of private issues. By the same token, the learner should not invite these discussions just because they are at a loss for words to make conversation outside of the office. This is a boundary we encounter in community-based practice and the learner will likely bump up against it during their rotation. More of this discussion occurs with the Rourkes' chapter (*see* Chapter 23) on relationships and boundaries.

Learners should be encouraged to join community events: hockey teams, knitting circles etc. This way they will feel more at home and experience some of the joy and balance which is vital to a successful rotation (and career) in a small community. This will usually need a bit of direction by the preceptor or clinic staff once the learner's interests are known.

Rural preceptors are role models in a broader sense for learners in a rural setting. That is partly because we model our behavior in and out of the office. They are likely to visit our homes and meet our families. We tacitly show how we have integrated personal and professional life while living in a small town. This allows the learner to make a more informed choice if this type of career is for them. Even if it is not, they will still face similar balancing tasks elsewhere in their career.

SCOPE OF PRACTICE

Rural rotations also show the unique integration of outpatient and inpatient care. Rural clinicians traditionally provide emergency room coverage as well as obstetrical care and inpatient management. It is invaluable to work with such generalists who, by necessity and disposition, wear several hats. This broad scope of practice may seem enticing to many learners – perhaps as much of a challenge as a more specialized career.

PRECEPTOR EXPERIENCE

Rural preceptors may receive as much as they give. For some rural preceptors, teaching may be the beginning of a relationship with the university department that may give career options as the relationship matures. Teaching may also prevent burnout and add interest to one's career along the way. As our students learn about our lives and practices, preceptors can take the opportunity to listen to their stories – particularly those learners from other cultures, who can teach us a lot about their path to medicine. Studies on the impact teaching has on community-based preceptors document increased enjoyment and keeping more up-to-date with evolving medical knowledge.

A 2001 survey in New England of 340 community-based preceptors noted 78% of them felt teaching helped them keep up-to-date medically and 75% believed it increased their enjoyment in their practice. They also valued the academic appointment they received. A similar Australian survey in 2005 found identical results as well as documenting the perceived intrinsic value of contributing to the students' knowledge and skill acquisition. In 1996, Chambers and Campbell surveyed 620 urban and rural British GPs to document their incidence of depression and anxiety. There was a statistically significant inverse association between mental health and participating in a teaching practice. In this study, clinical supervising appears protective of one's mental health.

There are other preceptor benefits. A key issue for many rural clinicians is that they almost always need to recruit new colleagues with whom to share the workload. As they age and wish to slow down and even retire, they would like to continue to live in their home community. Welcoming the next generation of physicians makes this possible. Retired rural physicians sometimes recount how they had to move away from their communities as patients needing medical care continued to seek them out despite their retirement, because of physician shortages.

MEDICAL MANPOWER

Rural manpower issues will affect education. There may come a tipping point where teaching capacity is reached. This will need to be determined locally. Changes in medical manpower add stress and workload to rural physicians who, at times, may need to lessen their teaching responsibilities or even take a break from teaching altogether. All this takes is one clinician to retire or move away to significantly alter the balance of work for the remaining clinical teachers. This delicate equation may need recalculation if one's clinical work increases as a result. Only the local practice can accurately decide this tipping point and their readiness to teach. Conversely, being a teaching site may attract like-minded physicians to join one's group. They likely perceive a teaching practice as a more dynamic work environment.

Preceptors often express concern about the time clinical supervision adds their day. Numerous studies in the USA in the late 1990s demonstrated that having medical students in one's practice was generally time and billing neutral. A recent set of studies in Australian community practices showed that the time taken supervising medical students was negligible if there was availability of a dedicated exam room for students and the preceptor joined the student and their patient at the 15-minute mark. This "parallel-booking system" is described in Chapter 9 on setting up a teaching practice. Ideally, it requires a spare exam room be set aside for the learner, so the preceptor could continue to see patients while the learner proceeds at a slower pace. On average, five minutes was added to the clinician's day in these primary-care settings. This study did not include any time spent in direct observation monitoring, chart reviews or discussion time at the end of the day. The highest estimated time referenced in the literature is an additional hour per day for precepting medical students. This might not be an onerous contribution to the profession, particularly if supported by the educational program.

COMMUNITY EXPERIENCE

Communities also benefit beyond recruitment of their future medical workforce. They receive significant economic stimulus, increased community enhancement and broaden the career opportunities and perspectives of their primary and secondary school students.

Rural high school students become exposed to medical students in their community. This provides them with role models, close to their age, for the first time. Arranging for the medical students to give presentations at local schools is a great experience for both parties, so that the circle can continue again from a new starting point.

The newest North American medical school, the Northern Ontario School of Medicine, opened in 2005. An economic impact study, several years later, documented that every dollar directly spent on the medical school promoted two dollars of indirect economic development. Attracting a two-to-one financial yield on such institutional investment in economically challenged regions of a country makes good public policy in the short- and long-term.

In northern British Columbia a medical school expanded into a four-year distributed campus in a northern region. A qualitative study, five years later, of interviews with key informants uncovered increases in civic pride, partnership development and community self-efficacy. This previously undocumented social capital is invaluable in remote areas traditionally tied to natural resource provision for their livelihood and community development.

UNIVERSITY EXPERIENCE

By participating in rural and remote education, expanding university medical programs are able to access training positions unavailable in the overtaxed urban centers. Beyond the saturation of these teaching hospitals, there is a developing acknowledgment that distributed medical education has great intrinsic value. The concerns around academic excellence have been put to rest as distributed medical undergraduate programs consistently score highly when tested against their peers. Rural medicine is gaining stature as both a geographic and vocational, if not cognitive branch of medicine. Internationally, rural medical journals produce unique insight into how healthcare is provided, when far from tertiary care centers.

Universities can develop important partnerships in the remote regions of their catchment area. Beyond sharing valuable educational expertise as faculty development, there is an obligation to develop wholesome professional relationships with rural clinical teachers. These clinical supervisors will need the acknowledgment and support of their professional and academic development.

Universities also need to develop relationships with these distributed communities. They share the political and social accountability mandate all government funders have to provide services to underserviced, typically rural and remote populations. We know very little about the health status of rural populations. Treatment protocols and triaging care plans are usually developed in urban centers with inherent assumptions of access to care and technology not generally available in small distant communities. Consequently, research opportunities abound in both understanding rural populations' health status and adapting treatment guidelines to remotely located patients. Such research possibilities can develop if important, respectful and even-handed partnerships exist between universities and cultural, social and political rural organizations. Universities need to acknowledge that they arrive, academic cap in hand. Although they have well-established roles in urban health science centers, they are strangers in rural and remote areas. They need to learn who the communities are and resist assumptions that they know any of the answers to rural issues. It may take years to even understand the questions. A new medical school in Northeast Pennsylvania took a creative research approach to listening to their communities. They led 23 community-based focus groups in 2010. They found out that most towns were very concerned with access to all types of medical care: preventive, primary, specialty and mental health services. The focus groups were the first step providing a connection between communities and the university, and have led to evolving partnerships.

SUMMARY

Universities bring essential curriculum, faculty development and evaluation tools to the community-based preceptor who can provide clinical supervision and teaching. Communities and patients provide the heart and soul of the whole educational experience, by allowing it to be integrated into their healthcare. University and community relationships, therefore, need to be respectful two-way relationships. Distributed medical educational placements have intrinsic value and are essentially different than hospital-based experiences, as our students are finding out. There is much to celebrate and little to fear.

FURTHER READING

Baldor R, Brooks W, Warfield M, *et al*. A survey of primary care physicians' perceptions and needs regarding the precepting of medical students in their offices. *Med Educ.* 2001; 35: 789–95.

Centre for Rural and Northern Health Research. *Economic Contributions of the Northern Ontario School of Medicine.* 10-A1. Sudbury Ontario: Laurentian University; 2010.

Chambers R, Campbell I. Anxiety and depression in general practitioners: associations with types of practice, fundholding, gender and other personal characteristics. *Fam Pract.* 1996; **13**(2): 170–3.

Garretson M, Walline V, Heisler J, *et al*. New medical school engages rural communities to conduct regional health assessment. *Fam Med.* 2010; **42**(10): 693–701.

Glasser M, Hunsacker M, Sweet K, *et al*. A comprehensive medical education program response to rural primary care needs. *Acad Med.* 2008; **83**(10): 952–61.

Hoat L, Wright E. Community-university partnership: key elements for improving field teaching in medical schools in Vietnam. *Rural Remote Health.* 2008; 4(4): 894.

Howe A. Patient-centred medicine through student-centred teaching: a student perspective on the key impacts of community-based learning in undergraduate medical education. *Med Educ.* 2001; **35**(7): 666–72.

Krupa L, Chan B. Canadian rural family medicine training programs. *Can Fam Phys.* 2005; **51**: 852–93.

Lovato C, Bates J, Hanlon N, *et al.* Evaluating distributed medical education: what are the community's expectations? *Med Educ.* 2009; **43**(5): 457–61.

Maley M, Worley P, Dent J. Using rural and remote settings in the undergraduate medical curriculum: AMEE guide no 47. *Med Teach.* 2009; **31**: 969–83.

Rosenblatt R, Hagopian A, Andrilla C, *et al.* Will rural medicine residency training survive? *Fam Med.* 2006; **38**(10): 705–11.

Rosenthal T. Outcomes of rural training tracks. *J Rural Health.* 2003; **16**(3): 213–16.

Rutter H, Herzberg J, Paice E. Stress in doctors and dentists who teach. *Med Educ.* 2002; **36**: 543–9.

Shannon S, Walker-Jeffreys M, Newbury J, *et al.* Rural clinician opinion on being a preceptor. *Rural Remote Health.* 2006; **6**(490): 1–13.

Strasser R. Community engagement: a key to successful rural clinical education. *Rural Remote Health.* 2010; **19**(1543): 1–7.

Strasser R, Hogenbirk J, Lewenberg M, *et al.* Starting rural, staying rural: how can we strengthen the pathway from rural upbringing to rural practice. *Aust J Rural Health.* 2010; **18**: 242–8.

Walters L, Worley P, Prideaux D, *et al.* The impact of medical students on rural general practitioner preceptors. *Educ Health.* 2005; **18**(3): 338–55.

Walters L, Worley P, Prideaux D, *et al.* Do consultations in rural general practice take more time when practitioners are precepting medical students? *Med Educ.* 2008; **42**: 69–73.

Worley P, Prideaux D, Strasser R, *et al.* What do medical students actually do on clinical rotations? *Med Teach.* 2004; **26**(7): 594–8.

15

Teaching in the Operating Room

John Dove

Many learners believe the operating room (OR) to be a place fraught with hazard, populated by surly surgeons, nasty nurses and laconic anesthetists. Like other challenging initiations, it is best to venture into such an environment with a guide.

For the clinical teacher the roles of guide, facilitator, and mentor to a learner can be rewarding. The potential effects of a good student learning experience in the OR range from the acquisition of good technical skills used appropriately, to career-changing realizations. The obverse is also true. Clinical practice in anesthesia and surgery has among the highest potentials for patient harm, as reflected in malpractice statistics, and physician premiums for malpractice insurance. How does one introduce a learner into this situation, while maintaining regard for patient safety?

An unfortunate reality of student rotations in many clinical situations is the "slotting" of students into schedules to "expose" them to various facets of medical practice. The duration of the scheduled exposure seems to be weighted according to the relative importance attached to that exposure by the student's supervisor or institution, and is often brief. How can the clinical teacher best assist the student to salvage a productive, appropriate and safe experience in a short time? I believe that the major tool is planning.

Rather than simply having the learner present to the OR on the first (or only!) morning of the scheduled rotation, the first step toward a successful outcome is communication between student and preceptor. In my clinical situation, as a family physician/anesthetist, in a small community, it was relatively easy to arrange a meeting with the learner before the first OR date. The discussion evolving from the following questions gives ample opportunity for the preceptor to create reasonable expectations as to what can be achieved in this environment, and using that information to establish an educational contract with the learner.

The questions are:
➤ What is the level of the student's education?
➤ Has the student had any prior OR experience?
➤ What is the planned duration of the OR experience?
➤ What are the student's goals for the experience? Are they realistic?
➤ Are there specific skill requirements that must be met by the learner and documented by the preceptor?
➤ How and when can learning be optimized?
➤ How much self-education is the student prepared to do?

Other specific issues that must be addressed are those of consent by the patient, patient safety, and feedback to the learner.

THE STUDENT'S LEVEL OF EDUCATION

Over the years, I have had the privilege of assisting many learners requesting clinical OR experience. Their qualifications have ranged from first year medical students seeking "real-world" rural medical exposure, to second year Family Medicine residents wondering whether to commit to a third year of residency training in anesthesia; to paramedics seeking to upgrade intubation skills.

Orientation to the OR environment is of prime importance. Explanation of the roles of various personnel is critical to the realization of our mutual interdependence as OR teams and is a cardinal point to be emphasized. The introduction of the learner to all members of the OR team should be done by the preceptor, and should clearly state the student's level of training, and the student's learning goals while in the OR. This is done to foster acceptance of the learner by the team; to enlist the support of the team for the student; and also to clarify what expectations may be reasonably be placed upon the student. I have found it helpful to request the assistance of the nursing staff to provide physical orientation to the OR; to describe the importance of and maintenance of sterile fields, and blood and body fluid precautions; and to teach scrubbing techniques according to institutional practices.

An early-phase medical student will benefit from the opportunity to become oriented to the OR; to see surgery and anesthesia in practice; and to learn certain technical skills, such as the starting of intravenous lines, under supervision. A latter-year medical student may be considering a career in anesthesia or surgery and often has questions about medical practice, in addition to acquiring clinical knowledge. The resident physician, who has already chosen a career path, may be seeking advanced airway skills, and increased knowledge about the pharmacology of conscious sedation, as examples.

THE STUDENT'S PRIOR OPERATING ROOM EXPERIENCE

The range of exposure to an operating environment among students varies tremendously. Today's medical student may have been yesterday's engineer, artist, NP or OR scrub nurse. We know that previous social and cultural experiences shape our responses to stressful and unusual situations. Certainly the student's first OR exposure is more likely to reveal unusual reactions, such as: functional dyspnea associated with the wearing of a surgical mask; claustrophobia associated with confinement in a darkened room, such as: during a laparoscopic procedure; and vasovagal attacks, such as during open bowel procedures, or amputations. Because of this and despite a surgeon's pressing need for an extra "pair of hands," the first OR exposure may not be good time for a medical student to become a *de facto* surgical assistant. The wise anesthesia preceptor elicits this information in advance, and enlists the support of the nursing staff to assist the student if necessary.

The Planned Duration of the Experience

Over the years I have had medical students and residents turn up on an OR morning and announce that they have been sent "here today to learn how to intubate." The cart is before the horse, likely because the horse has an obstructed airway. I like to discuss the "can't intubate, can't ventilate" scenario, and emphasize that intubation is but one facet of a skill set that comprises airway management. And if "that morning" is all that we have, airway management is what we will start to do. The learner can be shown techniques of bag–mask ventilation and given the opportunities to practice, to fail and to modify. From this, he or she is offered two salient points: first, that airway management is more difficult than it looks; and second, that the patient bears the consequences of an adverse outcome. I also offer additional time in the OR to allow opportunity to practice more bag and mask ventilation, the use of a laryngeal mask airway, and some intubation techniques.

This rests in contrast to the students who have a realistic amount of time to learn certain anesthesia skills. For these latter students, goals can be agreed upon which may include several techniques of airway management, the performance of lumbar punctures (aka spinal anesthesia), and the placement of central lines, as examples.

The Student's Goals: Are They Realistic?

The goals of the institution or program may not be realistic, but those of the student must be. One of the most important facets of the preliminary discussion is that it helps to align the preceptor and the student into a functional learning dyad. Components of this discussion must include many factors. The student's level of interest is important: is the purpose of this exposure for experience, the acquisition of a skill set, or a career choice? How much time will the student devote to this experience – one day, one week, one month? Are there performance expectations – such as an early-phase medical student, or a Family Practice resident working in an emergency room, might have.

Specific Skill Requirements

Flight paramedics and advance-care ambulance paramedics sometimes arrive as learners into the OR and have specific skill requirements. They are required to successfully perform a number of intubations, with safe and appropriate technique. The supervising anesthetist is responsible for documentation of numbers and assessment of technique. Medical students and residents have different requirements for evaluation, which should be discussed at the preliminary meeting or, at latest, on the first day of the rotation, so that planned and appropriate learning experiences can be arranged.

How and When can Learning be Optimized?

The practice of anesthesia is significantly procedural. Many of those procedures require continuing performance to maintain competence and minimize complications. Yet the "when" and "why" of choosing procedures or techniques require a knowledge base that involves the patient's medical status, the planned surgical procedure, and academic background. Learners frequently approach procedural knowledge by directing reading around the technical skills: the indications, contraindications, complications and benefits of a procedure, arriving latterly at the consideration of the patient. As the skill level of the learner increases, the role of the preceptor should evolve from that of physician who has selected the procedure, and aided the learner in its performance, to that of the physician who provokes the discussion about risks and benefits for the patient and management issues. This can be aided by case presentations, literature reviews, and non-judgmental challenges to the learner with a view to stimulating consideration of options. Both preceptor and student benefit from this interchange.

The Self-education of the Student

This facet of student education has long presented a challenge. As the performance of anesthesia seems to be based in procedures, the learning goals of most students are skill-directed, rather than academic. Recognition of this was highlighted in the publication of a text titled "Anesthesia for the Uninterested" by Birch and Tolmie in 1976.

I have found it helpful to refer students to an anatomy text with the request that they bring photocopies of the relevant anatomical diagrams to the OR, so that we can sketch what we see, diagram the landmarks and discuss our findings. This brief learning intervention, applied to each procedure, helps the student to understand what is being done, and why particular approaches are used, or avoided. As well, specific review articles are useful to give context to the procedures.

Another issue is the duration of exposure to the OR environment. Unless the student is undertaking a specific rotation in, or is committed to a number of days' exposure to anesthesia, learning will be fragmentary. This minimizes feedback, and impairs consolidation of knowledge.

CONSENT

The community hospital in which I have worked is known as a community teaching site, as part of the distributed learning model. Learners at various stages, and of several professions, have been present for many years; the published mandate of the hospital includes medical education; and the hospital consent forms for general admission, and those for surgical procedures, make specific reference to the presence of learners, and their participation in patient care. While there is general knowledge in the community that "young doctors" will be involved in hospital and clinic care of patients, the procedural nature of anesthesia, and the potential risks warrant specific introduction of the learner to each patient. As I provide a specific overview of the anesthesia procedure and risks to each patient, I state that the learner will be "assisting me" with the provision of anesthesia. Occasionally, a patient declines procedural consent for the learner. I reassure the learner not to take that personally. Since I will be doing the intubation in this case and the student only observing, I use this opportunity for demonstration of different anesthetic techniques which we might not otherwise cover: laryngeal airways, glidescope, etc. If the presence and involvement of a learner in the OR environment is unusual in your community setting, specific understanding and consent should be sought from the patient. Written acknowledgment would seem wise.

PATIENT SAFETY AND FEEDBACK

These are intimately related. The preceptor remains responsible for the actions of the learner. As all anesthetic procedures involve risk, supervision must be direct and feedback timely. The student must understand the necessity of ceasing an action immediately when told to do so, and withdrawing from the field if safe parameters are being broached (such as declining oxygen saturations during intubation) or when there is potential for trauma resulting from procedural difficulty. Each failure should be reviewed at an appropriate time as a goal-directed learning experience, in a non-judgmental fashion. It is useful to highlight the preceptor's own response to the difficulty of a procedure: some are intrinsically more difficult due to anatomic variation. The preceptor must be aware of patient status: teaching is important, but conversation should not interfere with the attentiveness required for constant surveillance of the patient under anesthesia. The deferral of discussion to a time when the preceptor's undivided attention can be given to the learner is safest.

SUMMARY

The OR can be a difficult venue for teaching due to the constrained, somewhat challenging, environment associated with the potential for high-risk consequences of failure. However, the risks are manageable, and the rewards are worthy. The preceptor has the opportunity to interact with bright, inquiring and usually enthusiastic students, and to aid them in the development of skills that can indeed save lives. It is very worthwhile.

FURTHER READING

Birch A, Tolmie J. *Anesthesia for the Uninterested*. Baltimore, MD: University Park Press; 1976.
Jeffree R, Clarke R. Ten tips for teaching in the theatre tearoom: shifting the focus from teaching to learning. *World J Surg*. 2010; **34**: 2518–23.

16

Teaching Procedures

David TS Barber and James Goertzen

Performing procedures is an enjoyable facet of primary care that allows physicians to hone another set of skills and change their day's pace. It also benefits patients, who receive more timely access to these primary care technical skills.

Regional specialists often feel burdened by performing simple procedures since this may delay their ability to perform the more complex procedures for which they were trained. In addition, continuity of care is also interrupted when a patient is referred out.

Performing lumps and bumps and other procedures presents a unique educational opportunity for the learner when placed in a community setting. The increasing average age of our patients, with its associated higher morbidity, swells the demand for procedures. It is critical that we train our physician/learners to be proficient in performing basic office procedures.

In this chapter, we will examine how the community physician can better train the learners in their practice, and look at tips to make this experience more rewarding for all involved. What we will discuss will pertain to office surgeries and procedures, although much can be applied to any procedure, including those in the emergency room and hospital. We will start by examining pre-procedure training, followed by tips during the procedure, follow-up care, and finish with complications.

PREPARING FOR A TEACHING PROCEDURE

When teaching a procedural skill, it is useful for the preceptor to have a sense of how we learn procedures. Fitts and Posner have articulated a three-stage model of motor skill acquisition (cognitive, integrative and autonomous) which provides useful teaching strategies.

Initially in the cognitive stage, the learner acquires an intellectual understanding of the procedure. Thus, the learner must have a conceptual understanding of the procedure before it can be performed. An important task of the preceptor is to deconstruct or break the procedure down into distinct steps.

This can be a challenge since the experienced preceptor who unconsciously performs the procedure may forget to articulate all the necessary steps. Preceptors can more effectively assist their learners during this stage by providing a chapter or short video to review, which demonstrates the procedure. As the learner initially attempts the procedure, they will consciously think of each step as it is somewhat mechanically performed. Learner performance of the procedure is quite variable and close supervision is required.

With practice and specific feedback, the learner solidifies their performance of the procedure and graduates to the integrative stage. Although the learner is still thinking about what they are doing, they are able to complete a procedure more fluidly with few interruptions and in a shorter period of time. During this stage, deliberate practice under the supervision of an experienced preceptor directs the learner to focus and perfect specific steps of the procedure. Unsupervised repetition of the procedure by the learner may solidify incorrect techniques.

As the learner gains experience with the procedure, they reach the autonomous stage. Their performance has become somewhat automatic and they can complete the procedure without thinking about separate steps. With their expertise, learners begin to adapt the procedure to different and more complex clinical situations where they may be required to vary their approach.

LEARNER SKILL LEVEL

The proceduralist teacher must prepare ahead to make sure that a teaching procedure is safe and effective for the patient, productive for the learner and efficient for practice. It is important to assess the capabilities of the learner, taking into account their previous experiences and level of training. For a learner with limited skills or experience, the teacher can work with the learner to help them practice the foundation procedural skills of sterile technique, handling surgical instruments, local anesthesia and basic suturing. The teacher also needs to reflect on what they are teaching: are they teaching the right skills, appropriate to the learner's level of training and procedural expertise?

Experience of the medical students can be divided into pre-clerkship and clerkship phases. Pre-clerkship medical students (generally first and second years) have very little exposure to even the basic procedures. Preceptors can provide these students with written or visual resources to review beforehand for procedures they may observe during the clinical rotation. Encouraging the student to practice the foundation procedural skills, in their own time, will allow the preceptor to more efficiently involve the student in specific steps of more complex procedures being completed. By clerkship, medical students will have at least done some practice suturing and, depending on their clinical opportunities, more advanced techniques and some other basic procedures (IV placement, ABGs, etc.). Hopefully, by the time the medical student graduates, they are gaining competence with basic techniques which they can build on during their postgraduate training.

Postgraduate residency programs usually have a list of procedural competencies they expect of their graduates. The community-based preceptor typically does all of these, or has a colleague with a slightly different practice which complements their own. Some programs require students and residents to track their procedural experience that has been shown to increase their involvement in procedural opportunities and accelerate their learning.

As the inclusion of IMGs into residency programs expands to meet the growing health demands of our population, their involvement has added much variability to the mix of residents' procedural competence and experience. Sometimes your resident has training as a general surgeon, in which case they can improve the preceptor's procedural competence; other times, the resident has a background as a pediatrician with little to no training/experience performing procedures and the preceptor may be required to focus on foundation and basic procedures.

There are many other ways that the teacher can assess the learner's experience and competency performing procedures. The easiest is to simply ask the learner what kinds of things they have done in the past and how comfortable they feel performing the procedure. With procedures that the learner may have opportunities to perform, the preceptor can better assess learner competence by asking them to describe and walk through the procedure from start to finish. One has to be wary of the cowboy mentality that sometimes exists with some students, who overstate their comfortableness and expertise with procedures.

PATIENT ASSESSMENT

It is good practice to ask the learner to assess the patient being considered for a procedure. The learner can then report their findings and procedural plan, giving the teacher a better indication of the learner's experience and confidence level. By developing a relationship with the specific patient, learner motivation and commitment to master the planned procedure is more likely to occur. Patients will also be more willing to involve the learner in completion of the planned procedure.

Practice and Simulation

If the learner has limited experience with some of the foundation and basic procedural skills, it is worthwhile to have them practice outside of the office. For integumentary procedures such as basic suturing or excision of lesions, one can obtain pigs' feet, which are readily available from the local supermarket, and some expired suture material is usually available from the nearest hospital. Sewing towels together may be a simple alternative, or practicing suture tying with string. Many suture kits are now disposable and the learner can use these usually discarded tools for practice. It is good practice to ensure that the learner has a solid understanding of the anatomy relevant to procedures. For scheduled procedures, the teacher can ask the learner to read up on the topic the day before and present the relevant anatomy. There are websites with 3D anatomy that may help the less visually inclined students.

An area of increasing sophistication and innovation is the simulation lab. These labs exist at many medical schools and allow the student to practice procedures in a simulated and realistic environment. The models used are interactive and can give feedback to the learner, going beyond the static anatomy models of the past. As an example, joint models that simulate joint injections let the learner know when the needle is in the correct anatomical space. These models are realistic and provide opportunities to practice a whole host of procedures. Most programs continue to develop their simulation labs, and it would be worthwhile to become familiar with this resource since, as a community-based teacher, you may have access to some of the models and other resources.

Keeping a "procedure box" around the clinic is a useful resource to develop. In this box or series of boxes, used equipment and materials can be stored for procedures that will be taught during the clinical rotation. This provides opportunities for the learner to handle spare speculums, needle drivers and trochars and get a feel for their weight and limitations.

Safety

Patient safety and satisfactory outcomes are common goals when a learner is involved in care. The proficient teacher is flexible in their approach to different procedures and recognizes that are many acceptable ways to perform the same procedure. One area where it is advisable to be less flexible and follow a more standard approach is with safety measures and universal precautions. Before the recognition of the methods of transmission of HIV and hepatitis, many physicians exhibited a somewhat cavalier approach to many of these safety measures. Although the experienced preceptor may rarely put themselves or patients at risk, a novice learner is more likely to accidentally incur a needle stick injury or cut themselves with surgical equipment. Most medical schools have provided students with clear protocols to follow in this area and as community preceptors it is important for us to follow these same protocols ourselves. If we follow "no touch or clean technique" for certain procedures such as joint injection, it is important that we have a collegial conversation with our learners discussing the rational for our approach.

Consent

Another area where a more standard approach is important is with obtaining and documenting informed consent for any performed procedure. The key to informed consent is a discussion with the patient where the procedure is explained, including rationale, risks, benefits and expected outcome. Although in most hospital settings, a written and witnessed consent is obtained, this is not a requirement for the office setting. What is essential to informed consent is a proper discussion with the patient and documentation that the discussion has occurred. Thus, many community preceptors will follow their informed discussion with the patient with a note in the patient's chart summarizing the discussion.

Indications and Contraindications

Fundamental to patient safety and the teaching of any procedure is that the learner acquires a thorough understanding of all absolute and relative indications and contraindications for a given procedure. Confirming a learner's competence usually requires a preceptor to review this prior to starting the procedure. If the learner has not mastered this knowledge, they can be directed to procedural textbooks for further review. It is also valuable to share the less discussed and more personal approaches of the preceptor. For instance, at what diameter of lesion or location one should consider referral to a surgeon or, what are the risks of removing lesions from different body sites and what body sites should one avoid performing excisions on. This may depend on the proceduralist's experience and local resources, but is important for the learner to be made aware of your limits. We usually share with learners five areas of the body to avoid: the temporal and mid-mandibular areas, the posterior triangle of the neck, the head of the fibula and the palm of the hand. Our rationale for this is the very superficial nature of the nerves (or tendons) in these areas, and their motor nerve components: respectively, the temporal and mandibular branches of the facial nerve, the spinal accessory nerve, the common peroneal nerve and palmar flexor tendons. The preceptor should aim to teach the learner to become aware of their limits and avoid getting into uncomfortable or unsafe situations. If the learner is uncomfortable with their level of competence for a procedure, they should consider referring to someone more experienced. Learners will find that, as they gain more experience, they will be able to take on what were once felt to be complex procedures.

THE PROCEDURE

The long-graduated physician quickly forgets how anxiety provoking performing a procedure can be. What is a now routine procedure for the experienced physician is seen as daunting by the learner. In this state of trepidation, the learner tends to omit some of the fundamental steps needed to ensure the anticipated outcome.

Positioning

Positioning of a patient can often be critical to how easily a procedure can be performed and, sometimes, even to its success. Learners, in their haste to get to the actual procedure, often give this step short shrift, which usually makes the procedure more difficult and the patient less comfortable. The learner, first, has to put the patient in a position that will be comfortable for the duration of the procedure and, second, to make sure that the patient position allows for comfortable access while performing the procedure. It is good practice to warn the learner about performing procedures on a patient sitting in a chair. While more efficient, there is always a risk a patient develops a vagal response and ends up on the floor. Surprisingly, this is more common with big burly males who are often unfamiliar with a doctor's office and disinclined to let you know that they are afraid of needles. It is important to teach the learner that, by spending a bit more time with this important preparatory step, they can make the whole procedure more efficient.

Pain

Learners tend to panic when causing the patient any discomfort, usually leading to more patient discomfort. While sometimes a bit more time-consuming, it is essential that the learner provide adequate anesthesia before starting a procedure. It helps the learner (and the patient!) through a procedure when the teacher has verified that adequate anesthesia has been attained.

Preceptor Limitations

Self-reflection is an important quality of the successful instructor of procedures and there are barriers to teaching that should be thought about from time to time.

Simplifying and breaking a procedure into discrete steps for a student is a common theme that the teacher needs to be aware of. When experienced at a procedure, it is very easy to lose sight of how complex that procedure really is. Instructors tend to dismiss or minimize their years of practice perfecting a procedure and, as a result, can expect too much from the learner. By underestimating a procedure's complexity, it is possible for the instructor to give too much responsibility to the learner, without adequate support. Most practicing physicians can cite examples of this from their own days as medical students: being left to repair a facial laceration in the ER on their own, or being left to remove a skin lesion with no one around to ask for guidance are just two examples. It is not appropriate for the learner or patient to be placed in a situation without adequate supervision and it is the preceptor's responsibility to ensure that the learner feels, and is, adequately experienced to perform the task at hand.

Variation of Approaches

The experienced instructor and proceduralist recognize the many different "right" approaches to managing lesions, closing incisions or injecting joints. However, over time we tend to limit our own approaches for reasons of efficiency or just personal preference and can sometimes be more dogmatic, and maybe less evidence-based, than we ought to be. When incorporating a learner into your practice it is important to reflect on this. Learners tend to be less overwhelmed by the number of ways available to deal with a lesion, than they are by the sometimes dogmatic approach taken by their instructors, especially when the student has experience with different approaches. For example, there are many suture techniques and materials that can be used to close an incision. At our local hospital, the surgeons all have their favorite suture technique and material that they swear by. Most orthopods have their favorite steroid that they inject into joints, but the evidence does not support one over the other. It is important for the learner then to recognize and appreciate the many right ways to approach performing a procedure. What they need to hear is the instructor's rationale for doing the procedure a certain way, and their opinion on risks of the alternative. The learner might appreciate you discussing other acceptable approaches and some flexibility or acknowledgment of alternative methods. One learns a lot from the enthusiastic students who have seen complementary approaches and are eager to share with, and be challenged by, their instructor.

Time and Effort

An area little discussed is how an instructor deals with the consequences of supervising a proceduralist in training: longer procedure time, often increased patient discomfort, and outcomes less ideal than had the instructor done it themselves. This is more challenging than supervising other aspects of patient care because, in the case of teaching procedures, the learner's impact on care is more tangible. In regards to patient discomfort, it helps to teach the learner proper techniques of anesthesia but, even then, the instructor needs to tolerate an acceptable level of patient discomfort: joint injections done by a learner will never be as slick as those done by the instructor. The instructor needs to develop a level of tolerance, and when beyond this, be ready to step in and take over. It is helpful to divide compromised outcomes into cosmetic or fundamental. For cosmetic, one has to develop tolerances for, and when beyond these, to consider revising. For fundamental outcomes (for example, full excision of a skin cancer or technique leading to a higher rate of infection) the instructor needs to have very little to zero tolerance.

Complications

Despite firm supervision, complications will arise, but one needs to accept that complications arise even when learners are not involved. There is also tolerance on the patients' part for small imperfections made by the learner. In academic settings, the patients are made aware that learners are always involved in their care and can choose to attend a non-teaching clinic. In the community setting, there are often fewer options for patients. It is important that the community teacher notify their patients of student participation in their care and, should they wish, give them the opportunity to have their procedure performed by the preceptor alone.

Complications are an inevitable consequence of performing procedures. Anyone, no matter how well trained or careful, will have to deal with a complication, whether it be a wound infection, wound dehiscence, or other. This is the most uncomfortable aspect to performing procedures, and probably one of the reasons why many primary care physicians shy away from procedures. The learner needs to understand that if they continue doing procedures, they will at some point have to deal with a complication. It is incumbent on the teacher to advise the learner how to best deal with these situations. In a post-procedure debriefing it might be worthwhile to explore with the learner how they would handle its potential complications. How would they handle a wound dehiscence or infection? New graduates tend to make certain mistakes when dealing with complications.

Pride often hinders the patient with complications from getting best care; it is difficult for the newer graduate to accept the complication, swallow their pride and refer to a colleague who may be better able to manage that complication. At the same time, one need not overdramatize the possible outcomes of a complication. For instance, although not ideal, wounds that have dehisced and heal by secondary intention generally look fine. Patients' expectations are more often than not less lofty than the physician's. Alternately, it is wise to avoid doing procedures on the patient who will accept nothing less than a perfect result, and to share these concerns with the learner.

The last area around complications that the instructor should explore with the learner is the evolution of the apology by the medical community. Over the last decade, it has become more acceptable to apologize to patients for less than perfect outcomes or complications from a procedure. It is important that the learner understand that by apologizing for a poor outcome or complication, one is not acknowledging wrongdoing or negligence. One is apologizing for a known complication of a procedure that should have already been acknowledged and accepted by the patient. By apologizing, the proceduralist removes barriers between themselves and the patient; this often leads to better understanding and a higher level of co-operation, engendering quicker resolution of the complication.

Follow-up Care

The learner should be expected to give the patient any post-operative instructions and answer any questions around expectations and follow-up. Ideally, the instructor also has hand-outs, as this will standardize patient instruction and help guide the learner. If possible, the learner's contact information should be given to the patient as first contact in case of complications or questions; the learner can better understand what type of questions, concerns or complications that they should anticipate in practice. Furthermore, it is good practice to book the patient for follow-up with the learner. This allows the learner to explore what the patient went through after the procedure, look at any visible results of the procedure, review any pathology and remove sutures. Sometimes, more learning occurs during the follow-up appointment than during the procedure itself. One can see how difficult removing sutures which were too small to begin with can be, or how a flimsy cast does not survive the follow-up interval!

SUMMARY

Performing procedures is a fun part of our practice, but teaching it requires us to share the fun. There may be times when we are better off just doing it ourselves if that is what we really want to do. Generally though, we need to have a standard approach of assessing the learner's capabilities easily and having a graded complexity and degree of supervision established. Our learner will be developing career-long habits and, if they are to follow our example, these should be safe and effective for patient and physician.

FURTHER READING

Dixon-Warren N. Competency scores of common procedural skills as self-reported by graduating family medicine residents in Ontario. In: *North Ontario Medical Program News*. Thunder Bay ON; 1997.

Fitts P, Posner M. *Human Performance*. Belmont, CA: Brooks and Cole; 1967.

Goertzen J. Learning procedural skills in family medicine residency. *Can Fam Phys*. 2006; 52: 622–3.

Hutten-Czapski P, Magee G, Wooton J, editors. *Manual of Rural Practice 2006*. Shawville, Quebec: Society of Rural Physicians of Canada; 2006.

Kelly L. Surgical skills for family physicians. *Can Fam Phys*. 1998; 44: 469–70.

Milne R. Minor surgery in general practice. *Br J Gen Prac*. 1990; 40: 175–7.

Rennick R, MacRae H. Medical education: teaching surgical skills – changes in the wind. *NEMJ*. 2006; 355(25): 2664–9.

Spike N, Veitch P. General practice procedural skills. *Aust Fam Phys*. 1991; 20: 1312–16.

Wearne S. Teaching procedural skills in general practice. *Aust Fam Phys*. 2011; 40(12): 63–7.

Websites

www.cfpc.ca/uploadedFiles/Education/Procedure%20Skills.pdf
www.cmpa-acpm.ca/cmpapd04/docs/resource_fils/ml_guides/consent_guide/pdf/
com_consent-e.pdf

Other

Anatomytv; Procedure consult; *NEJM* clinical video series.

17

Teaching Preventive Care

Karen Hall Barber

When faced with an eager medical learner in the office, one tries to formulate a mental checklist of skills to impart to the undergraduate or postgraduate trainee. In doing so, one typically includes appropriate procedures or exam techniques such as how to distinguish a benign pediatric murmur from one that is not, inject a joint, examine a frightened child or perform a comfortable pap smear. Where does teaching preventive care fit in? Most of us instinctively incorporate it efficiently into our practice, based on years of experience. It seems somewhat amorphous and difficult to conceptualize, let alone nurture as a skill in a novice who is perhaps more concerned with concrete knowledge gaps such as antibiotic coverage or titration of insulin. This chapter will articulate what it is that we do as practitioners when we address this less tangible yet vital area within family medicine, and give some tools and references for your teaching toolbox.

APPROACH TO PREVENTIVE CARE IN COMMUNITY-BASED MEDICINE

Unlike other disciplines within medicine, one of the cornerstones of family medicine is that we have a cohort of patients that we call our own and care for long-term. When it comes to preventive care, as their primary care physician, we are responsible to this entire roster of patients when they come into our office and perhaps even when they do not. Thus, we differentiate two categories of preventive care when we consider where it is that we offer an intervention. Preventive care is addressed either in the office or through a cohort-based proactive recall initiative.

In the office, we either look after preventive care *en bloc* during a dedicated, more thorough appointment such as at a periodic health examination, or we try to intervene opportunistically, on the fly so to speak, when patients come in ostensibly for other reasons. Alternatively, when considering how to attend to preventive care within an entire practice, we use wide and varied approaches for trying to keep track of due dates of various interventions and fashion recall processes to update them. Sometimes, we defer to external partners such as public health. Some of us run dedicated clinics such as an influenza campaign to capture a greater number of patients. Sometimes at these dedicated clinics, we also target other initiatives; for example, we complete additional required immunizations along with reminders for mammograms at an influenza vaccine clinic, thus targeting as many topics as possible to as many patients as possible.

Teaching Preventive Care

Medical knowledge is expanding and sometimes it is hard to stay on top. Should we add "teaching preventive care" to medical learners on top of their ever-growing foundational requirements? How do we translate what we know about the skilled application of preventive care into an effective learning experience for the student in our office? Attention to preventive care is typically a part of accreditation for postgraduate programs. Finding a deadly disease at an early stage can decrease morbidity and mortality and can be critical incidents for the patient and the physician. Smoking cessation counseling, tedious as it may be, is a more worthwhile use of our time than palliating a patient with the resultant lung cancer. So, yes, preventive care is an important part of our practice and, therefore, also of community-based medical education.

Including the topic of preventive care as a teaching objective for medical learners who come through our practice is a win-win endeavor. It gives one the opportunity to reflect on how one's own practice is fairing with respect to preventive healthcare. With a learner in the midst, there will be the opportunity to get a fresh set of eyes on current practices, typically with practical suggestions. Moreover, the additional hands "on deck" in your practice might allow for an effective proactive roster-wide preventive care intervention to be executed (depending on the duration of time that a learner is in your practice and what their other responsibilities and time commitments are).

If their rotation with us is long enough, learners will gain experience in each of the following areas: locating applicable resources, critical analysis of preventive care guidelines, application of preventive care with individual patients, how to adapt preventive care interventions when necessary, application of prevention care with wider cohorts of patients, and understanding effective identification of patients in need of particular preventive care interventions by having a thorough approach. One looks at this list of learning objectives and recognizes that they are tiered, based on gaining foundational experience from the bottom up. In this regard, if the student is in our practice for a shorter period of time, perhaps they will gain experience in only the bottom few tiers of the pyramid. If they have a longer rotation with us, consider mutually agreeing upon ways in which the student can gain experience in each of the preventive care teaching tiers by assigning appropriate preventive care projects. Figure 17.1 gives an overview of five teaching point tiers within the realm of preventive care.

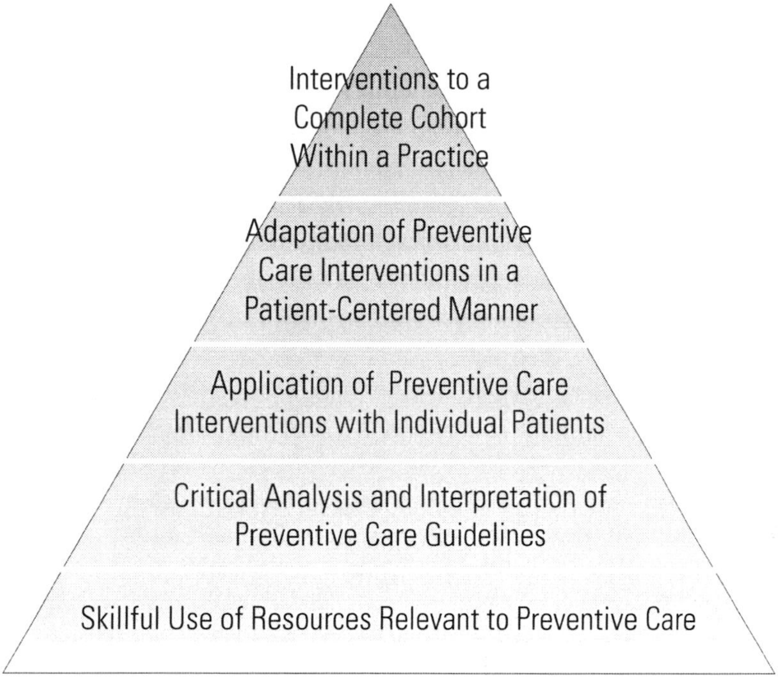

Figure 17.1 Preventive Care: Tiered Educational Objectives

1 Resources

Learning about the plethora of available prevention care guidelines, and how to deftly locate appropriate recommendations on topics one is not familiar with, is one of the first educational steps. We recognize this as the foundation upon which we base all of our preventive care interventions: one must first be familiar with the guidelines as a starting point. A preceptor can initiate this during a case or chart review by incorporating topical questions such as "What do the osteoporosis guidelines recommend in this particular patient demographic?" If one gets blank stares in response, the next task is to direct the student to look up the corresponding guidelines, giving them time to do so, and report back their findings to you for further discussion. (Perhaps your practice has rapid access to internet resources and, if so, this discussion can take place on the fly quite quickly. If your practice is not set up with internet, perhaps this task will be set aside for researching after clinic.) If one gets a long dissertation from the learner about what the guidelines say, then advance the questioning to teaching point 2.

Physician Resources

In our respective medical jurisdictions, we each have efficiency tools that help guide us and cover more ground effectively during periodic health examinations. For example, the College of Family Physicians in Canada endorses and allows for PDF printing of these commonly used, evidence-based and peer reviewed tools: *The Rourke Baby Guide* for newborns to 5 years of age, *The Grieg Health Record* for 6–17-year-old patients, and the *Preventive Care Checklist Forms* to guide us with adults' general assessment visits. If you do not currently use one of these tools in your practice, it might be a beneficial exercise to task your student to locate and trial appropriate forms with your patients and provide feedback on their utility or lack thereof. As is often the case, learners often bring new resources to our clinics and our patients.

Patient Hand-outs

Next, assist your student in gaining experience with locating effective and appropriate hand-outs for patients. Depending on your practice, setting up this might involve asking the student to find an existing hand-out or pamphlet on a given subject or, better yet, create his or her own. Your learner will also want to gain experience in being a resource to the patients by connecting them to pertinent community resources available to them. Many medical learners are adept at accessing and printing online resources for patients, to give at appointments or demonstrations to patients in the exam room (if office set-up permits). How to navigate to an especially helpful patient website such as the American Lung Association's online program for smoking cessation or directing a new mom to appropriate web-based community resources can be helpful for computer-savvy patients. Your learners very likely will be able to show you helpful links that you were not previously aware of. Consider assigning your learner a show-and-tell style "lunch and learn" session demonstrating various resources they have found particularly helpful during their rotation. It is important to have reliable and appropriate websites for patients, to offset the plethora of advertising-based information on the internet.

Interprofessional Collaboration

Lastly, under the category of resources, direct your learner to be mindful of acquiring the skill of being able to tap into resources that involve people rather than limiting "resources" to functional tools. Consider tasking your student to seek out and learn about manpower types of resources that may be available to the practice or patient to improve the effectiveness of preventive care interventions. These might include collaborative preventive care initiatives with local hospitals or public health, NPs, dieticians, pharmacists or other community supports. Not uncommonly, when having a student in the office, one learns about resources or services that were not previously in your preventive care toolkit.

2 Critical Analysis and Interpretation of Preventive Care Guidelines

One aspect of preventive care guidelines that one should encourage a learner to gain familiarity with is the different classification systems that describe strength

of evidence behind given various preventive care recommendations. This is easily covered by asking questions around this topic during a case discussion. If a
57-year-old man is in the office for a periodic health examination, a vigorous
discussion could ensue around the strength of evidence surrounding prostate
cancer screening. One might ask "What is the strength of evidence behind this
particular preventive care topic, and how does that compare to other topics?"
Given that preventive care guideline are dynamic entities and thus continu-
ally changing over time, be mindful, as a teacher, that our own practice styles
or protocols which address various preventive care initiatives may very well
be out-of-date. As such, be prepared and open to accept challenge and suggestion from the learner in your practice. Again, learning from our students,
consider giving them an assignment to present your team with the current recommended practice guidelines for given preventive care initiative. Be prepared
to learn!

The next level of awareness relating to preventive care guidelines is to familiarize oneself with the situation that occurs when two or more medical entities
present misaligned preventative care recommendations. The recommendations around colorectal cancer screening, as advised by the Gastroenterological
Society of Australia, may not be entirely aligned with what the Royal Australian College of General Practitioners recommends. One could ask the student
something like, "Given that two different medical groups have their own disparate recommendations, which guideline is most applicable in this situation?"
or which ones are most aligned with the principles of family medicine and
local community resources.

The last suggestion within this teaching point is to guide your medical
learner to scrutinize preventive care recommendations with an eye to identify
peer-reviewed guidelines without industry influence. This can be accomplished
through case discussion, by assignment or perhaps a continuing medical education group that regularly meets to review various topics in family medicine.
In this latter setting, it can be effective to then choose a topic for the group that
is appropriate for the student and learn alongside them.

3 Application of Preventive Care Interventions with Individual Patients

When we offer an in-office preventive care intervention, it is either at a dedicated office visit that is geared towards addressing these items *en bloc* or one
devises various reminders or prompts to add on a preventive intervention to a
visit that was booked for something else. These both are essential skills to show
our learners.

We need to share with our learner, explicitly and by example, the many ways
that "opportunistic" preventive care can be achieved. Some possible ideas are
having the student fashion waiting room appointment checklists that are spe-
cially designed to prompt a patient to self-identify a needed maneuver such as

an overdue tetanus shot, mammogram, FOBT or similar. For example, "Please help us keep you up-to-date by telling us if you think you are due for an immunization, blood work or pap smear."

Building on this in-office deployment of needed preventive care interventions, one needs to then further develop efficiencies when administering more than one preventive care intervention in a given office visit – i.e., find how to maximize preventive care interventions without jeopardizing time management. Time management is an area that learners often struggle with, and it can be troublesome to direct a learner to both maximize preventive care interventions and also improve their time management! This may involve encouraging your student to think about how to identify, ahead of the appointment, what initiatives are needed through a chart pre-review. Or to liaise with the front staff or a nurse to help one create systems and or medical directives that will allow for preventive care maneuvers to be more automated.

4 Adaptation of Preventive Care Interventions in a Patient-Centered Manner

Continuing up the pyramid of tiered objectives, the next skill is the adaptation and deviation from preventive care recommendations in a patient-centered manner. A brief joint "pre-appointment patient chart preview" discussion targeted towards patients that you know require an adapted version of a preventive intervention can be a powerful learning experience. For example, you know that 45-year-old Mrs. Smith who has the 11 o'clock appointment has a first-degree relative with colon cancer from age 50. You might ask your learner to specifically pre-read that chart and tell you in what way the preventive care guidelines should be modified in this situation.

Alternatively, you are going to want to direct your student to paying special attention to patients you know will be somewhat difficult to successfully negotiate a specific intervention. For example, you know that 35-year-old Mr. Jones booked in at 10 o'clock is coming in because he just read a magazine article about colon cancer and that he told the receptionist that he wanted to have a colonoscopy. Or Mrs. Chen who is wary of every preventive care intervention you routinely offer her. These guided interactions on your part will help your student gain experience in negotiation and partnering with patients when recommending preventive care interventions.

And lastly, we want to reinforce with our learners that the key to effective identification of which patients are in need of what particular preventive care interventions is to have a thorough approach. We want to impart to our learners that obtaining a complete past medical/surgical/procedure history, family history, medication list, allergy history, functional inquiry, lifestyle review and clinical examination is an important tool that we have to use for effective preventive care. You might be able to effectively demonstrate this point if you notice a situation when the student overlooks or misses a key family history item with a patient, such as their mother and sister had breast cancer, that might have changed the preventive care recommendation. Obviously, having a charting system that highlights preventive care hallmarks is optimal. Most electronic medical records are easily adapted to this function.

5 Application of Preventive Care Interventions to a Complete Cohort Within a Practice

The top tier of the preventive care objectives is the one that pulls it all together. Fully addressing this category might have to be reserved for situations when a learner is in your practice for an extended period of time, or in a more advanced level learner. Selecting *which* topic to address for a cohort-based preventive care initiative is a skill worth working on with the learner in your practice. It is important to find common ground when trying to marry the interests or passions with your student with the current priorities for your practice. For example, you and your learner might negotiate that the student will do a base-line clinical audit in your practice with an aim to make recommendations to improve the number of patients who are successfully covered by their initiative. But the topic or project the student chooses has to be one which is valuable to both of you. The learning will be more meaningful if the student has a sense that their hard work will impart real and tangible change to the practice and improve patient care. Consider a situation where a student has a plan to do a baseline audit to identify which patients need to be taking additional vitamin supplements but this is not a particular initiative that you are likely to take up in the long-run and sustain. Therefore, the hard work that the student puts in will be for naught and likely this will be perceptible to the learner. Spend some time up-front negotiating a topic that is aligned with the preventive care goals that you have for your practice and that the student is interested in. For example, you might have a suspicion that you could improve on percentage of 2-year-olds who have completed their baby immunizations. This is a topic that the student is also interested in, therefore, the overall project will be far more successful with respect to having sustained gains for your practice and be a meaningful learning experience for the student. Once the topic has been determined, further refining it into a clinical question with hypothesis is the next step. The key is to keep it crisp and focused. One might narrow it to tackle varicella vaccines. The question might be "Were all eligible children in my practice born after 2006 immunized with varicella?"

Picking the topic and clinical question is perhaps the easy part. Next, you will have to work with your student to explore ways of identifying the relevant cohort of patients that are to be captured in the preventive care initiative. If one has a fairly robust electronic medical record, one might be able to identify the specific cohort with relative ease. Barring that, one might have to get creative and expect more manual data extraction. Once the cohort is identified, performing a clinical audit is the next step. One of the key learning points from a clinical audit is to reflect on the next steps. "I have the data, now what do I do with it?" One then determines if the clinical question was answered but, more importantly, what does it mean? You might have found that 14% of eligible children did not receive varicella vaccination. Literature reviews would help one interpret the meaning of the 14% and what the unvaccinated rate should be. Hypotheses might be proposed as to why some children were missed. Suppose one determines that a rate of 14% of eligible children being left unvaccinated is not your practice goal; further observations and proposals need to be made to try to determine why some children were missed and how to get the future rates higher and how to identify the children who were missed to revisit the topic. When this last cohort is identified, one needs to be mindful that there may be some children who have contraindications or parents who declined the vaccination in the first place.

The most exciting part for the learner is to use all of the information gathered, thus far, to devise and possibly implement steps to remedy the deficit and plan for improvement going forward.

SUMMARY

Teaching preventive care to medical learners is perhaps a previously underemphasized yet essential area to highlight during a community-based rotation. To do this well, one needs to first review one's own approaches within your practices and then teach the tiered preventive care objectives using this same lens. There are innumerable rewards from having a medical learner in your office; not least of these are the benefits reaped by your patients from having fresh approaches to an often overlooked area within your practice.

FURTHER READING

Primary Care Toolkit for Family Physicians, Rourke Baby Guide, Grieg Health Record, Preventive Care Checklist Forms: Available at: www.cfpc.ca (accessed August 9, 2011).

18

Teaching Care of the Elderly

David TS Barber

Medical care of the elderly in a community-based setting requires a different tempo and set of skills. Typically, the busy practitioner enters a slightly altered timeframe when seeing an older patient. One changes one's interactions, interpretations and care planning with this patient group. We will review some of these basic concepts that a teacher needs to convey to learners in the care of the elderly.

In larger academic settings specialty-trained geriatricians often consult on or follow complex elderly patients whereas in smaller communities this specialty is not readily accessible and is not generally required for most aged patients. Elderly living in smaller communities are managed by generalist family physicians even as their care becomes more complex or transitions into a long-term care (LTC) facility. In rural communities, telehealth consultations with geriatricians may be available for complex cases where pseudo-dementia, cognitive impairment and psychiatric issues may overlap or where aberrant behaviors are making caregiving very challenging or unsafe. Otherwise, generalist care in the norm.

One of the main differences between teaching students in an academic versus community setting is that there is more emphasis on making sure that the interaction between the teacher and learner does not interfere with efficiency and productivity of the clinical practice. One has to take into account the number of available rooms that the community practice has and the patient load per day. More importantly, the proficiency of the learner will determine their efficiency; a learner who might be struggling with foundational clinical skills can feel overwhelmed when they are now asked to adapt these newly-acquired skills to an aged population. This can easily clog up the flow of an office. These issues are not as important in academic settings, where ideally, the offices and schedules and remuneration have taken the impact of learners into account.

AMBULATORY CARE

Office Appointments

Generally, the elderly person presenting to the office is more complex than a younger patient. The geriatric patient has more health issues, medications, questions, and preventative health needs. It is important to give the learner a sense of the "real world" regarding appointment intervals (i.e. relatively short-time slots), but some flexibility might help the learner on their way to synthesizing data. To help the inexperienced learner (medical student), it is worthwhile giving them a time limit, and reviewing the patient with them beforehand to help focus the visit. Without guidance, it would not be unusual for the inexperienced learner to spend an hour with a patient. It might also be useful for your practice and the medical student to review and update a patient's medication or problem list. The more experienced resident should require less guidance and be much more independent and adept when seeing these complex patients.

Continuity

Depending on how long a learner is spending in your practice, there is great benefit to continuity of care, especially with elderly patients. It allows the learner to follow-up on and evaluate any changes to medications or care plans that they might have recommended. More importantly, continuity fosters a therapeutic relationship between the learner and the older patient, which is often the most rewarding part of providing care to this population. It is, therefore, useful to instruct your office staff to try and book follow-up appointments with the same learner.

Patient Context

Patient context is much more important in this demographic than other sectors of medicine. Missing that a 40-year-old patient lives alone is far less important than not recognizing or documenting the same for an elderly person. It is recommended that when learners see elderly patients, they become familiar with the patients' home situation, daily activities, social supports and family involvement. Creating a space for this documentation with an electronic medical record (EMR) or paper chart is helpful in guiding your learner.

Learning About Available Community Supports

An idea to help a learner give better care is to charge them with learning about appropriate community supports for the elderly. There will be an expectation in the future to have the elderly live at home for far longer than in the past. The only way that this is going to be feasible is for the healthcare provider to have an intimate understanding of how to utilize these community resources to the advantage of keeping the senior living in their own home. Possibly, your learner might discover some resources that you were unaware of.

Keeping an Eye on the Learner: Different Models of Observation

There is a debate within the academic settings about the best model to balance learning with observation. Should the preceptor be seeing patients in parallel with the learner, or be focused only on the learners, and not seeing patients? This has led to variability across academic teaching sites. Some sites have a "resident only" group of patients: these are seen only by the learners and never see a staff physician. The oversight of this group needs to be fairly strict, with live video or direct observation of the interactions as the norm. The other end of the spectrum has a group of patients shared by preceptor and learners. Generally, the residents in this situation are more independent and are directly observed less frequently. This model is mostly used in the community setting for two reasons: there is no pre-existing video feed and community physicians are not often compensated for their teaching, thus there is an expectation for the resident to "earn" their experience by helping the physician see patients in parallel.

In the context of seeing elderly patients, this presents challenges for the overseeing physician and presents risks to the elderly patient population. Depending on the stage of the learner, varying degrees of close initial observation are warranted, and there are a few areas to be vigilant. Residents prescribing medications for the elderly generally have difficulty accepting the maxim "start low, and go slow" and if inexperienced in prescribing, may not heed this advice. Another area within the prescription arena that needs close oversight is category of medication used. It is important to instill within the learner a degree of respect for relative higher potency of drugs within this age group and to be especially wary of medications known to problematic (for example, NSAIDs, narcotics, medications with anticholinergic properties, etc.). It might be useful to have the new learner review all new medications they have prescribed until you are comfortable with their ability to prescribe safely to this population.

Biological Versus Chronological Age

A community physician knows that the health of the elderly population is quite varied. It can be difficult to engender to learners that work-up, treatment and preventative care might be vastly different in patients of the same chronological age. Young learners tend to think dogmatically, where everything is black and white, where rules are to be followed and there is only one proper technique. This is a probably a product of their undergraduate training, where success requires the understanding of the right answer. Especially when treating the elderly population, it is important to modify the early learners' rigid thinking. One obvious area is having them explore the importance of biological versus chronological age and life expectancy. We have all seen the extraordinarily fit 80-year-old with a possible life expectancy of another 20 years. This is in contrast to the 80-year-old with oxygen-dependent COPD, diabetes and coronary artery disease with possible life expectancy of only a few years. The learner initially has difficulty accepting that these two 80-year-old patients will be managed in completely different ways with respect to work-up of disorders, preventative screening and treatments. This is a great opportunity to explore with the student how aging tends to tilt the risks/benefits balance of testing, treating and preventative screening towards risk and away from the benefit as one ages.

Similarly, existing guidelines need to be malleable and the learner needs to learn and accept this subtlety of medicine. For example, current guidelines may recommend screening for breast cancer starting at the age of 50 and stopping at 74. One has to look at the patients' biological age and life-expectancy before applying these guidelines, in which case, it might be reasonable to stop screening in one patient at the age of 60 while in another case, one might continue screening to 80 and beyond.

The Concept of the Frail Elderly Person

This is a very useful concept for the learner to become aware of, and can be used across the continuum of care of the elderly. The experienced community preceptor learns to be cautious of pigeon-holing patients, as this sometimes leads to misdiagnosis or enables confirmation bias. However, in this situation, categorizing a patient as a frail individual can be helpful for a number of reasons, and is an easy concept for a learner to understand. Although no clear definition exists for this sub-population, it is meant to identify the elderly patient at higher risk of disease or injury. These are patients who are close to the tipping point of illness. It is important for the learner to recognize these patients because they are always more sensitive to the common illnesses of the elderly, and often manifest disease in atypical ways. For example, a viral URTI in the healthy elderly may be of typical presentation, while, in the frail elderly, this can present with delirium. One needs to be in tune with this condition, and interpret presentations differently, as well as modifying treatments. Preventative care for this population also needs to be modified. One needs to pay close attention to the frail elderly's support network and, if insufficient, to make sure that as many community supports as possible are put into place.

Illness in the Elderly

Certain topics are best not taught didactically, rather to be learned through experience. One of these areas is the varying presentation of illness in the elderly. There are a few important points that should be emphasized with the learners early on, while they have access to teachers. It is accepted that one must always balance the risk of therapy versus its benefits. We know, for instance, that when giving a patient a prescription of indomethacin for gout we accept (and inform the patient) that the benefit of the drug must be balanced with the risks of the taking the medication. The physician prescribes the medication and the patient takes the medication because it is assumed that the benefit therapeutically outweighs the risk of potential side-effects. What the learner must recognize is that in the elderly, the risks tend to increase, sometimes so much that one may need to alter therapy or consider another therapy altogether. In the case of NSAIDS, we need to teach the students that the risks of taking this class of medication is much higher in the elderly and one should consider modifying its use (lower starting dose, shorter course, addition of proton pump inhibitor), check for contraindications (borderline renal function, patient on ACE inhibitors with diuretic), or alternate therapy (local steroid injection, colchicine in the case of gout). The inexperienced learner will frequently take what they have learned from adult medicine and apply to the geriatric population, without taking into account a shift in the risk/benefit equation. The community preceptor needs to guard against this.

The use of investigations should also be modified when working up an elderly person's condition. Many students will aggressively and indiscriminately work-up all conditions without asking the question "What will I do with the results?" or "How will this change management?" For instance, in the elderly with sciatica, is it appropriate to order an MRI of the spine? To help determine the appropriateness of any study, the student should first ask himself or herself what they would do with a positive finding. Given an elderly patient's biological age, state of health or advance directives, the recommended intervention (disc surgery in this case) leading from an investigation (MRI) might not be feasible, safe or consistent with a patient's directives. As patients age, the value added by diagnostic testing needs to be questioned more often, and the increasing risks of testing justified. This issue is even more relevant in the long-term care population and will be addressed in a later section.

Just as there are no rules about stopping screening procedures, the same applies to medications used for primary and secondary prevention. We do not know when to stop statins, or many other common preventive pharmaceuticals. Common sense may dictate simplifying medication regimes as our patients grow older and frailer than the population for which they were originally intended. This will be a new skill for the learner who has invested most of their energy to this point in learning how to initiate medications!

PREVENTIVE CARE IN THE ELDERLY

As primary care physicians, we place great emphasis on preventative care measures for our population. Most of a learner's knowledge of this topic comes from standard screening guidelines. What is usually missing from the guidelines, however, is when to stop screening, which becomes more relevant as patients age. Also, there are preventative measures unique to the elderly population that the learner should be aware of.

There are no hard rules about when to stop screening and this area falls more into the "art of medicine." Taking into account a patient's life-expectancy, the aggressiveness of the condition being screened, the risk of the screening measure itself and the risk of further investigations leading from a positive screen (false or true positive), the experienced physician can make a judgment as to the appropriateness of a screening measure. For example, it is hard to justify screening for colon cancer by fecal occult blood testing in an 85-year-old with multiple co-morbidities.

One also needs to consider adding other screening modalities for the aging patient. To prevent falls, the learner needs to consider screenings for vision, hearing, mobility and poly-pharmacy. Having the student review all of an elderly patient's medications is a great way for the student to learn pharmacotherapy and can highlight how the aging body can alter a drug's pharmcokinetics and effects. This would be a good opportunity for the student to familiarize themselves with the Beers Criteria and the rationale for medications being on that list. And when the student recommends that your 85-year-old female taking nightly lorazepam for past 45 years should stop taking it, this will open up a nice discussion about the risks and benefits of stopping medications, and possibly the benefits of the therapeutic relationship.

The student should also consider driving assessments when seeing elderly patients. The learner needs to be aware of their responsibility around mandatory reporting and driving ability of patients.

OTHER FEATURES UNIQUE TO THE OFFICE ENCOUNTER WITH THE ELDERLY

Patients are very effective at covering up early cognitive deficiencies and it would be a rare family physician who has not been duped into thinking that a moderately demented patient is of sound mind. A human's ability to confabulate and fill in blank memories is truly remarkable. Sometimes, it is the spouse who raises the issue of memory or a family member contacts the family doctor with concerns. Sometimes the nurse picks up on some odd behavior. The learner needs to understand the subtleties of dementia and potential clues that might lead to identifying the condition early. The standard measurement of cognition still seems to be the Mini-Mental Status Exam (MMSE), although more students are being taught to use the Montreal Cognitive Assessment (MoCA), while Mini-Cog and Clock Drawing test are also validated and commonly used. While some in academic centers might advocate the need to regularly screen individuals for dementia above a certain age, this is usually impractical and likely unnecessary in the busy community practice. The preceptor should emphasize to the learner the need to be alert to the possibility of early dementia in the elderly patient and to be quick to screen with the appropriate test when needed. The learner will appreciate your tips on how to introduce this test without making the patient (and themselves) feel uncomfortable.

LONG-TERM CARE

The LTC home is a great place for the learner to explore and hone their skills caring for the elderly population. Most communities have at least one LTC home and the preceptor should see that the learner is introduced to this environment. One of the first impressions most clinicians and learners have is the typical odor associated with many such facilities. Rather than have occasional unpleasant experiences, there is value in regular visits to see the positive aspects of the patients' lives and the dedication caregivers provide to those in their care.

Our family medicine department in Kingston, Ontario has begun a pilot project in which each supervised resident is responsible for the care of 10 LTC patients for one year. They are expected to take all calls from the home, make any emergency visits for their patients, perform quarterly drug reviews, and lead family conferences. An on-going study is measuring the impact of this program on the learners' competence caring for the LTC patient and any impact this may have on their decision to practice in LTC upon graduating.

There are many benefits to getting learners into the LTC setting, some obvious and some less so. The spectrum and complexity of disease is quite wide in LTC homes and is a nice way to introduce the learner to many of the common diseases in a more relaxed, less rushed setting. The learner appreciates the atmosphere of independence and feels empowered in this setting. Over time, they start to appreciate the relationship they develop with the residents of the home, which, as those who take on this challenge know, is the most rewarding part of this area of medicine.

CARE OF THE ELDERLY IN THE EMERGENCY DEPARTMENT

When the geriatric patient suffers a marked decline and is seen emergently, the interrelatedness of function, physiology and cognition described above takes on a more pressing dimension and gravity.

The clinical teacher in a busy urban emergency department will commonly see ill or confused geriatric patients. The clinical scenario may be quite different in a small community hospital where the elderly patient may be well-known to the emergency physician or the nurses. They can often spot a change in pre-morbid functional or cognitive level of the patient, since they know the patient. This sets different levels of clinical challenges but certain lessons affect the teaching of care of the elderly in the emergency department:

➤ elderly patients often present atypically – one always needs to think "outside the box"

➤ the clinician and learner will be unlikely to be able to focus on just one problem – these are complex patients with multiple chronic problems

➤ both functional and cognitive assessments must be factored into management and diagnosis.

Learners in a busy emergency department will be frustrated by the older complex patient. The student will likely need some orientation to the three Ds of cognitive impairment: depression, delirium and dementia. They may need some reading resources before the rotation begins. They will need to have access to some of the simple, quick cognitive assessment tools available: the six-item screener for cognitive impairment; the identification of seniors-at-risk tool; and depression screening methods. The clinical teacher knows that delirium, while less common than depression or dementia, is associated with high mortality rates. Rather than seeing the confused and confusing geriatric patients as "social admissions," the ground work for distinguishing among the three Ds should be laid.

Broadly inclusive medical work-up, careful medication review and collaborative information from family members are all part of the learning curve for caring for these patients. Since the diagnosis may be unclear even after hospital admission, having the learner follow such admitted patients is an excellent learning experience.

Focused care of the elderly in the emergency department is a developing subspecialty within emergency medicine in urban centers. Smaller community hospitals will benefit from prior knowledge of the patient, but the learner will likely not share in this. These will, therefore, always be challenging cases for learners, who may need both additional direction and supervision.

SUMMARY

Care of the elderly certainly broadens the scope of care and, if managing patients at a LTC site, can get us out of the office, which is often refreshing in itself. Beyond the widened scope and environment of practice, one begins to appreciate the relationships with the elderly for many reasons: often they are more ill and engender more sympathy; or, their life experiences or wisdom resonates with you; or, they are mellower and have more realistic expectations of care. For the younger physician, these qualities are often hard to appreciate in the busy, hectic years of building a practice and raising a family, but they become more salient over time.

Care of the elderly requires a gentle touch and a patient mind. Teaching it and introducing learners to this delicate set of patients also needs to be thoughtfully conveyed to our learners. Learners that do best in this environment are those who can empathize, not just sympathize, with the elderly. With empathy comes the understanding of the often unique suffering of an elderly person; for example, nocturia and the challenges of getting out of bed and into the bathroom safely in the middle of the night. Beyond empathy, those learners who quickly appreciate and respect the unique physiology of the elderly person is better able to manage their health needs. The learners that I worry about, and keep my eye on, are those who are not seemingly overwhelmed by the demands of this age group; the good learners initially struggle with complexities of the age group, whereas weaker learners may tend to ignore them.

FURTHER READING

Centre for Studies in Aging & Health at Providence Care resources. Available at: www.sagelink.ca (accessed August 9, 2011).

Daichun L, Van Brussel L, Hansen K, *et al.* But I see old people everywhere: dispelling the myth that eldercare is learned in nongeriatric clerkships. *Acad Med.* 2010; **85**(7): 1221–8.

Fick D, Cooper J, Wade W, *et al.* Updating the Beer's criteria for potentially inappropriate medication use in older adults: results of a US consensus panel of experts. *Arch Intern Med.* 2003; **163**: 2716–24. Available at: www.archinte.ama-assn.org/cgi/content/full/163/22/2716 (accessed August 9, 2011).

Geriatric Resource Guide from Northwestern University. Available at: www.galter.northwestern.edu/geriatrics/ (accessed August 9, 2011).

Ismail Z, Rajji T, Shulman K. Brief cognitive screening instruments: an update. *Int J Geriatr Psychiatry.* 2010; **25**(2): 111–20.

Prendergast H, Jurvich D, Edison M, *et al.* Preparing the front line for the increase in the aging population; geriatric curriculum development for an emergency medicine residency program. *J Emerg Med.* 2010; **38**(3): 386–92.

Samaras N, Chevalley T, Samaras D, *et al.* Older patients in the emergency department: a review. *Ann Emerg Med.* 2010; **56**(3): 261–9.

Towards Optimized Practice: Available at: www.topalbertdoctors.org/infomed_practice/clinical_practice_guidelines.html (accessed August 9, 2011).

Unwin B, Spoelhof G, Porvaznik M. Nursing home care: part I. Principles and pitfalls of practice. *Am Fam Phys.* 2010; **81**(10): 1219–27.

Unwin B, Spoelhof G, Porvaznik M. Nursing home care: part II. Clinical aspects. *Am Fam Phys.* 2010; **81**(10): 1229–37.

19

Palliative Care

Len Kelly

This is one of the most creative aspects of healthcare. Nowhere is the art and science of medicine so clearly on the surface. The art involves listening to the patient and their family. The science includes the basic medicine of the physiology and pharmacology of disease process and pain and symptom management. The creativity comes in simplifying the pharmacology – so that even family members can administer oral or subcutaneous medication without worry or guilt, and steadily navigate changing emotions when they are caring at the home for a dying family member.

A CARING FOCUS

Palliative care requires all the healthcare team to change focus. We are not reversing a disease process, or fighting infection to restore a previous level of health. Primary care physicians notice the change when they leave a busy office to do a palliative care home visit. The rush of the scheduled day must be put aside, we must slow down. Sometimes it is like taking stock, a deep breath, as if entering a church. We are stepping into a different time zone, a reality in which everything takes on more meaning: words, smiles, humor, pain, fear. As Ian McWhinney recalled: "Talking to the dying showed me that we shy away from asking about fears, when often the fears are quite specific: 'Will I have pain? Will I suffocate?'" (Reproduced from the *Canadian Journal of Rural Medicine*; 1998; 3(3): 168–9, with permission).

There is nothing typical about end-of-life caregiving. It affects the clinical teacher. They may have known the patient for decades. How will a learner fit into this sometimes confusing and spiritual aspect of primary care? Many people die at home at their request, but most die in hospital. These are quite different settings. One is very private, very personal, and shared with the family. The other is a more clinical setting with help and input from the nurses and support staff, who also have many other duties to attend to.

I try to let the learner know several things about visiting a dying patient.

We begin with some clinical background of how we arrived here, then a picture of the patient, their character and their family dynamics. I point out that stressful events like this sometimes bring out difficult family dynamics and we may be faced with just that. Anger is sometimes directed toward the medical team. "Why wasn't something done sooner? Why can't you fix this? Are you just going to let them die?" It can change daily. Often, there is great peace and room for humor. Always there is the need to address comfort needs, answer questions and listen. A chaplain colleague pointed out to me: if someone talks to you, sit and listen; if someone holds you hard or weeps on your shoulder, these are silent words. Listen, enter into the pain, and wait.

ROLE-MODELING

After orienting the learner, we visit the patient. I always introduce the learner to those present, but do not expect much conversation from the learner unless started by the patient or family. I have prepared the learner with the second part of the orientation: that we are not in charge, we are here to help out. We ask the patient how they are, how are the caregivers doing that day, any practical issues: pain, caregiver fatigue. As a clinician, I try to focus on finding the "vibe," the undercurrent. When the patient seems comfortable and there is a sense of peace, I tell the caregivers that this is what we want – i.e. that it doesn't get any better than this. This helps us all have similar goals and re-orient unrealistic ones. This tells family members and the learner that the goal is a peaceful setting, where pain is controlled, even at the expense of an alert patient.

After we leave the patient's home, I often simply pause and take a deep breath. I ask the learner how they felt and if they had any questions. The debriefing is on two levels: how are they feeling – fear, peaceful, nervous? They may have a personal perspective based on experience of losses in their family. It is our role to listen to these reflections. Asking if they have any questions allows us to see where they might be at. If they ask about practical issues – use of subcutaneous morphine, clinical complexities – these are great learning opportunities for clinical content. It also tells us that they might not be dealing with this at an emotional level, and that is fine. They do not need to experience what their teacher does. If their questions are about more psychosocial issues then we spend time on those questions.

The practical issue about palliative care is that it is time-consuming. I usually have a second physician involved, so that if I am unavailable, someone else is. This is particularly necessary if the course will be lengthy or if I will be away. Similarly, the student will not always be able or willing to attend. The student can learn a lot at the time of pronouncement of death – but they also cannot be available 24/7 and may miss it. Be sure to let them know when you see them next about the death if it occurs in their absence. Do not expect the news to have any particular emotional impact on the learner, as they are not as connected to the situation as you likely are.

The teaching of palliative care is more about role-modeling, doing less rather than more. Despite the need of some of our medical knowledge, our presence needs to de-medicalize dying. Because of this, it may take us out of our typical comfort zone. Some learners do very well with it and others appear disinterested. Either response is fine as long as they are respectful. Learning about palliative care is a career-long study. Students who do not like it or feel uncomfortable with it can often avoid it, in their eventual practice. But it is important to model respectful humility, which is a very different role than we assume as team leader, say, in an emergency room resuscitation.

Before going into a home or hospital room to declare someone deceased, I tell the learner what we will do. We will go in and approach the patient, listen with a stethoscope for absent heart beat and then say a neutral statement, such as "they are at peace now," or "their suffering is over" or "you are right, they are gone." Stroking the patient's hair and holding their hand is a form of respect, then, we back off to let the family get closer if they wish. The learner sees the quietness involved; the neutrality of the statement. Some families like to thank you, some are overwhelmed. It is good to step outside and give them time.

Again a deep breath may be in order. You can model quietness with the learner as well. If you or they shed a tear, that is fine. Talking about it adds little, but the learner may have some questions or comments. After the paperwork is completed and we are leaving the home or hospital ward, I always thank the learner for their help. Often their quiet presence is their only contribution – but they have seen one way of doing palliative care.

It is not all gnashing of teeth; the smile of a dying patient is very infectious. Often family members are ready for some humorous recounting of past family events. I am no longer surprised by the belly laughs which can arise for some of these interactions. We can follow the family's lead and enjoy it!

There is some science to good palliative care and it is good to have some articles on hand for the reflective or inquisitive learner. It is, however, a deep well of experiential learning, often accessed later in one's practice. So, the expectation of the learner is to observe and participate in a small way. An experienced learner may do their own patient visit if they are comfortable. There is no definitive way of proceeding beyond pain control, relationships and respect (*see* Table 19.1). The penny may drop years later when the learner is palliating their own patients and recalls some of their learning experiences. Think of it as an investment in the learner which includes a degree of self-disclosure by the clinical teacher.

Table 19.1 Teaching Palliative Care

Orient the learner to:	Patient character
	Family dynamics
	Objectives for the visit
Debrief:	Re: emotional experience
	Re: clinical questions
Expect:	To teach by role-modeling
	A wide range of learner reactions, includes "disinterest"
	This is a long-term "investment" in the learner

EMOTIONS

One's own sense of mortality will affect end-of-life teaching, learning and patient care. Martin Donohoe, an Oregon physician, suggests sharing literary selections about dying from physician-authors. He saw this as a way of sharing the breadth of emotions a clinical teacher or learner might experience. He incorporated brief readings into discussions of critical incidents or read at rounds. Topics include:

Sharing grief: Lewis Thomas's "The Young Scientist," the intern crying while presenting a case at morbidity and mortality rounds.

Anxiety: William Carlos Williams in "Danse Pseudomacabre": "How can a man live in the face of this uncertainty? How can man not go mad with grief, with apprehension?" ("Danse Pseudomacabre" by William Carlos Williams, from *The Collected Stories of William Carlos Williams*, copyright © 1938 by William Carlos Williams. Reprinted by permission of New Directions Publishing Corp.)

Acceptance: Somerset Maugham's "Sanitorium:" "I don't mind dying any more. I don't think death's very important as love." (Reproduced from *The Complete Short Stories of Somerset Maugham*, with permission of AP Watt Ltd on behalf of the Royal Literary Fund).

Osler, often quoted as saying that if he wasn't humming or whistling, he'd have been crying upon leaving the room of a dying patient.

These and other literary sources of emotional experiences by physicians can normalize the range and intensity learners (and their supervisors) may experience during caregiving during end-of-life care.

ATTITUDE

A longitudinal postgraduate experience in Israel showed positive attitudinal (and skill) achievement when residents were given shared responsibility for a patient receiving palliative care at home. As part of an interdisciplinary team, with their physician supervisor, they were responsible for weekly home visits and team meetings and two-weekly didactic sessions on specific topics. After 8 months requiring 3 hours per week, they felt this longitudinal exposure to interdisciplinary palliative care helped them accept the philosophy of care inherent in end-of-life care:

➤ the futility of aggressive life-prolonging measures
➤ acceptance of death as an outcome
➤ a focus on alleviating suffering
➤ ability to prepare the patient and family for the inevitable.

Their measured attitudinal changes included lowering barriers to using morphine and were accompanied by specific skill and knowledge development.

EDUCATIONAL INITIATIVES

A 2003 US study of residents in Connecticut by Schulman-Green documented that most participants learned by their own experiences and by making mistakes. They also showed significant physician anxiety in dealing with dying patients. One resident commented "You do far too much learning by making mistakes." (copyright: Institut Universitaire de Gériatrie de Montréal). These house staff were also greatly influenced by the attitude and behavior of their attending.

This set up the dynamics of highly teachable moments: anxious, ill-prepared learners open to direction and learning. If observing their supervisor was an effective way of learning, then the behavior and attitude of the clinical teacher must be a powerful determinant of their experience of end-of-life caregiving. These are likely unrecognized critical learning moments and need to be acknowledged as such. This also identifies the need for some debriefing and checking on how the learner is affected by such experiences: "How did that feel? Any thoughts or comments?" (*see* Table 19.2)

There is a need for effective formal teaching and integration of palliative care into a broad scope of coursework. When learning about congestive heart failure, sepsis or cancer, a significant part of the clinical teacher's experience will involve the care of dying patients, but that is rarely integrated into the disease topic:

➤ What symptoms does a patient dying of end-stage heart failure experience and how are they best managed?
➤ How conscious is the dying patient with septic shock and how do we manage that aspect of their care?
➤ How do we understand their care wishes?

These questions recognize the losses in which all disease processes culminate. Some might call this treatment failure, but is still end-of-life care. These end-events have likely challenged the clinical teacher over the years and may be worth sharing as disease management is discussed. What is amenable to instruction is pronouncement of death. Short workshops on what to say, what not to say and how to apport oneself have been shown to help residents practically and emotionally deal with dying patients and their families. Pre-death communication reinforces for the resident, and the family, that the patient is gravely ill, even if they suffer from a potentially recoverable disorder. Role-playing in such workshops allows for practicing respectful methods in a safe environment.

Table 19.2 Approaches to Teaching Palliative Care

➤ Integrate end-of-life care into disease-specific education
➤ Adopt a multi-faceted approach to resident training: communication skills, knowledge, attitude, comfort level
➤ Role-modeling is very important
➤ Recognize the intensity of clinical experience may supersede the length of a rotation
➤ Understand that the default outcome is that the resident will learn by making mistakes

DESIGNING POSTGRADUATE PALLIATIVE TRAINING

The art of designing effective training in palliative care is a developing one. The appropriate length and format of curriculum is difficult to conclude from the evaluation of existing programs. Systematic reviews of North American postgraduate training initiatives demonstrate sub-optimal outcome assessment, usually without control groups. The outcomes generally measured were four-fold: communication skills, knowledge, attitude and comfort/confidence levels. These reviews demonstrated that communication skills are best enhanced by using role-playing or simulated patients in two-hour (or longer) palliative care workshops. Brief didactic sessions showed objective improvements in focused knowledge areas. Relevant length of clinical rotations was less clear. Rotations from two weeks to longitudinal one-year experiences all had positive, but poorly measured, effects. These reviews suggest a shift from traditional time-based clinical rotations to a multi-faceted approach might be optimal. This would include interactive sessions for communication skills and focused didactic sessions on symptom management, use of opiates and hospice care criteria. They also noted that the positive effect of the clinical experience may be most related to the intensity of the experience rather than the length of the rotation – leaving this an academic challenge, as well as a highly individual learning experience.

SUMMARY

Palliative care education and care provision continues to evolve in scope and approach. What remains unchanging is the need for committed clinical teachers to role-model effective end-of-life care. This may take place in an evolving educational milieu but will always need a degree of self-awareness, fearlessness and respect on the part of both the teacher and learner.

FURTHER READING

Bickel-Swenson D. End of life training in U.S. medical schools: a systematic review. *J Palliat Care.* 2007; **10**: 229–35.

Donohoe M. Reflections of physician-authors on death: literary selections appropriate for teaching rounds. *J Palliat Med.* 2002; **5**(6): 843–8.

Kelly L, O'Driscoll T. The occasional palliative care patient: lessons we have learned. *Can J Rural Med.* 2004; **9**(4): 253–6.

Marchand L, Kushner K. Death pronouncements: using the teachable moment in end-of-life care residency training. *J Palliat Med.* 2004; **7**(1): 80–4.

Schulman-Green D. How do physicians learn to provide palliative care? *J Palliat Care.* 2003; **19**(4): 246–52.

Shaw E, Marshall D, Howard M, *et al.* A systematic review of postgraduate palliative care curricula. *J Palliat Care.* 2010; **13**(9): 1091–108.

Sinclair S. Impact of death and dying on the personal lives and practices of palliative and hospice care professionals. *CMAJ.* 2011; **183**(2): 180–7.

Singer Y, Carmel S. Teaching end of life care to family medicine residents – what do they learn? *Med. Teach.* 2009; **31**: e47–50.

20

Research

Len Kelly

For most clinical teachers, an interest in research is a developmental stage in their career. The first 5–10 years are professionally consumed by the practicalities of establishing a practice and a family/personal life and work balance. Once a clinician is settled into practice, there is energy for reflecting on and questioning one's clinical management, established disease recommendations and deepening one's understandings of day-to-day illnesses, which might prompt research interests.

Further training in doing research is an excellent option for those who can pry the time away from clinical work. If that is not possible, collaborating with those who have such expertise makes sense.

Several years ago, I wrote of the *"10 commandments of community-based research."* These signposts may be useful for the community-based clinician who takes on doing some research:

1 *Curiosity*: We become more curious as we age. If we are well-informed and a question does not have an apparent answer, this is a "researchable moment." Raise the question, see if it has been answered.
2 *Question*: Write down the question; discuss it with your learners and colleagues. Is it a topic which needs qualitative or quantitative methods? Many clinical questions can be answered with relatively small sample sizes of fewer than 100 participants.
3 *Literature search:* A basic search will often tell you if your question has already been answered, but perhaps the population studied differs from your patients. Does what is out there satisfy you? Is the literature search and review you have written substantial enough for publication on its own?
4 *Write the title:* This is a simple but very important step. Using a minimum of words forces us to focus our language and thinking. Look at the title, is it doable? The nouns will often be the outcomes and the adjectives the variables. You are now moving along in the research process. Now you

can take the idea further in discussions with colleagues, because you have clarified exactly what you are asking.

5 *Collaborate appropriately:* This means that you seek out colleagues who know more about the topic than you do; hopefully, they are also more experienced in research. It does not mean that you are the source of community-based data for someone else's ideas. But if that is your role, then it still deserves full partnership in the research project, including authorship. This is also where involving a learner can instill energy into the project. Offer authorship to all colleagues who offer help and will stay involved throughout the project. Collaborating may also take the form of creating or joining a network of similar-minded clinicians.

6 *Ethics:* Assume that any research initiative requires approval by an ethics board. You may not know of them, but all universities have them, as do many regulatory colleges. This needs to be done before any data are gathered and is often quite off-putting. Research boards often use inaccessible language, as they are typically set up for more invasive and controversial issues than you are proposing. You may well need assistance with this task.

7 *Data gathering:* Not quite like picking wildflowers I'm afraid. In small community practices, there is a power differential between the patient and physician and this may preclude many topics, or require that the interviewers are unknown third parties. There are also cross-purposes: the patient did not come to the clinic to participate in research, they came for medical care and attention. That said, your clinic staff can be invaluable in getting consent, handing out surveys or collecting chart information. EMRs make some of this much simpler.

8 *Analysis:* Consult a statistician rather than a therapist here. Always discuss the project with an interested statistician before you gather any data. Offer them shared authorship and listen to their advice on how and what data need to be acquired. Manually filling out information or having to pull charts a second time usually means that there was a disconnect early on. This can really limit what questions can be answered.

9 *Write-up:* Start writing with a firm template. Get the template from a likely journal to which you will submit. Even if you are not sure where you will send the article, adopt an established template. Journal articles have become shorter due to decreased advertising support, and concise writing is very important. Using "instructions for authors" will also help keep you from omitting uninteresting, but required, sections like "methods."

10 *Rewrite, resubmit:* Your article will likely be rejected. You will not be prepared for this, but it will happen. It is important to look at the expert comments made about the rejection. Use these for rewriting the paper and making it stronger. Consider resubmitting to the same journal or elsewhere.

The seven deadly sins are:

1 *Not protecting enough time:* You have to protect a morning or afternoon that you will regularly set aside for scholarly work, otherwise it will never get done. Sometime on-call shifts can give you some opportunities for getting work done. If you cannot set aside any time at this point in your career, then put off any interest in research till a later time. You might consider writing down your thoughts and ideas for later processing.

2 *Not asking for help:* Get help before you expend too much energy hitting your head against the wall. Research is like any skill: you may come by it naturally, but more likely you will need some help along the way.

3 *Not listening to the help:* Experienced researchers may point out that you have bitten off more than you can chew. Listen to them. There may be methodological or practical issues: access to enough patients, geographic limitations. Being realistic early on is very wise.

4 *Thinking the research is not important because you are frustrated or tire of it:* Stay the course. If you thought it was a good idea before you encountered hurdles, it still is. Once you have a sense of what the project involves, you may decide that it is not for you, or that you will need help with it.

5 *Thinking you are not up to it:* It is inevitable that, at busy times, the project will sit and gather dust. It is harder to get back into it once you have left it for a while. Major roadblocks may be not having enough time or needing more collaboration.

6 *Trying to cover too much:* What will it take to prove or highlight your point? Would a well-written letter to the editor suffice where a research project may not be feasible?

7 *Not finishing:* Dust it off. Get help. Choose some time when you can take another run at it. Pare it down, go into salvage mode. Does the literature review have enough merit on its own?

The three virtues of research:

1 *Increased confidence:* You are a scientist as well as a clinician and teacher: Why else would you think in a questioning and critical manner? Research broadens your sense of professionalism.

2 *Increased professional and academic standing*: Research is one of the many ways to contribute to the profession; this may be a good fit for you.

3 *Less untilled fertile ground*: If medical writing or research is something you always wanted to do, then take some simple steps to accomplish it. Shorten your professional bucket list.

Research is a vast field which can be very intimidating. How do we get there if we want to? Considering a graduate degree is one of the surest routes. Many Master's degrees are now given by distant education and can be done from your home, but they are very time-consuming. More practical for many would be dedicated research courses designed precisely for a busy clinician. Start small and move forward and set aside the time and energy you will need; that will be the tricky part.

QUANTITATIVE AND QUALITATIVE RESEARCH

Quantitative research investigates the quantities of measurable items: doses, effects and probabilities. Qualitative research measures the qualities of experiences: emotions, attitudes and feelings. While these two streams represent different philosophical traditions and assumptions about reality, qualitative and quantitative are both important ways of researching in medicine. Qualitative methods will be a better fit for understanding social and personal realities. Quantitative methods will continue to serve us well in scientific inquiry into the biomedical and statistical world. One will help us understand feelings and thoughts; the other, biochemical and biological realities. Different questions beg different methods (*see* Figure 20.1).

Both methods are indirectly very familiar to us. We use applied research every day in our office. When we ask a patient how they are feeling, we are following a qualitative line of understanding. When we measure blood pressure response to the initiation of a new medication, we are looking at a quantita-

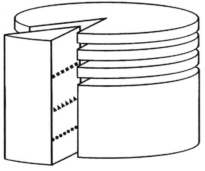

Quantitative Research:
thin layer of generalizable data

"Thin" data (looking at one element) over a large area (large sample size) which might apply to a large population. Objectively it is designed for a broad perspective and generalizablility.

Qualitative Research:
thick slice of data, not generalizable

Rich, "thick" personalized information which might not apply in all places (for all individuals). But, you can get at layers which quantitative methods may miss (e.g. a survey which might miss something important). It results in subjectively processed data but may be the only way to access this highly personal information.

Figure 20.1 It All Depends How We Slice the Cake

tive (n=1) experiment. Generally, the "hard" research of quantitative methods is more highly valued than the "soft" data uncovered by qualitative methods. This is a reflection of socio-historical movements arising from the positivist tradition. The "reality is objective" perspective historically gave rise to many offspring: freedom from religious predominance, support for the technological revolution and development science: biology to microbiology, physics to the study of synapses (*see* Figure 20.2).

Because qualitative methods are such a good fit for primary care questions, we shall spend some time discussing this option. Quantitative inquiry is very systematic and likely needs to be learned in an apprenticeship arrangement with a more experienced researcher. Even though it avoids the complexity of statistics, it is a very rigorous methodology. Some of the philosophical and structural differences between qualitative and quantitative research are outlined below.

QUANTITATIVE RESEARCH

Quantitative research is more familiar to us than qualitative. Our practices may change by the results of large randomized controlled studies or meta-analyses of groups of them. The range of their influence is in the number. The number of participants, the "p" value, the number of variables studied, the number of subjects. Their influence depend on their findings, the size of the study and on how similar their participants are to our patients.

At the bottom of the heap is the "n of one," a case report. Clinicians can be very affected by single critical incidents, especially if the outcome is poor. From a research perspective, these incidents and other, less onerous, but interesting cases can be very informative. Getting these cases published is becoming more uncommon. Publishers tend toward printing prospective studies with a healthy sized cohort followed over time or randomized controlled trials (RCTs).

Chart reviews (retrospective observational studies) can be very informative. They can tell us about the diseases we are seeing in our practice and how we are managing them. This is much simpler if electronic records exist, but often management questions will require going to the chart. Since this can be very time-consuming, involving a medical student who has a research requirement is ideal. From an educational perspective, having a learner pull even 10 charts on a given topic will give them a research experience which is simple, but provides them with a valuable overview perspective.

Surveys are the classic entry-level quantitative study and these can be done with the help of one's office staff. There is an art to designing a good survey and they typically need three or four drafts and a trial run before they can move forward.

Participating in primary care networks to add a small number of subjects to a large multi-centered trial is another option if the question is of interest to the clinician.

Quantitative Research

Theory

▶ A quantity
– an experiment measuring effect
– a survey tabulating numbers

▶ Measurable outcomes

Assumes reality is distinct from observer and is measurable. Positivism tradition ("the world positively and objectively exists"). It uses scientific method: hypothesis, testing and measuring to learn about the world.

Deductive
Objective
– generalizable, "thin" data
– measurable outcomes:
  dose/effect, causality, percentages
  "How angry is subject?"
  "How often does it occur?"

Qualitative Research

Interview data

▶ Interacting with subjects and interpreting their responses and feelings
– the qualities of their experiences

▶ Themes, understanding

Assumes reality is a series of relationships which includes the researcher. The tradition is called interpretive (hermeneutic), in which we discover relationships as we study them. We understand the world as a series of events which individuals experience uniquely; we try to understand the quality of that experience.

Inductive
Subjective
– non-generalizable, "rich" data
– leads to understanding deeper human elements:
  feelings, attitudes
  "How do you feel?"
  "Why are you angry?"

Figure 20.2 Qualitative and Quantitative Theories of Research

Literature reviews on in-depth topics can also be an entry into research activities. Recently, journals prefer systematic reviews which impose rigorous critical appraisal standards to the literature being reviewed. These are generally quite a reach for the novice researcher but not out of the question.

Presenting one's research can include a poster presentation at a conference one is planning to attend, or scripting a letter to the editor or an opinion or artistic piece for a journal.

Levels of Evidence

Bear in mind in reading and contemplating research, there are standard categories of how powerful the type of study is. The levels do not ensure that the study has been well done but gives a sense of the standards the research must meet.

There are three similar standards by which the level of evidence of a study is categorized. The most widely used is the American:

Level I: RCT findings (including meta-analyses and systematic review of RCTs)

Level II: other well-designed studies

Level III: expert opinion

Australian levels of evidence are:

Level I: systematic review of RCTs

Level II: a single RCT

Level III: other well-designed studies

Level IV: case series

Level V: this level is often unofficially added for expert opinion

The UK NHS uses an alphabetical system:

Level A: RCT or cohort study

Level B: Retrospective, case-controlled studies

Level C: Case series

Level D: expert opinion

These levels of evidence give clinical researchers a hierarchy approaching scientific "truth." Community based physicians can use this as a scoring system of how solid the evidence is and, combined with a collateral level of recommendation stratification, can decide if the study and its recommendations are reliable. The next question is whether it applies to their own patient population and is relevant to their practice. Community-based clinical researchers may be involved in a regional or network RCT, but are more likely to participate in level II studies. In quantitative research, the practice of critical appraisal allows one to see if the study lived up to its standard and if it might apply to your patients. Qualitative studies (generally considered level II) are assessed by different measures of accuracy and validity.

QUALITATIVE RESEARCH

Qualitative research is defined by both its methods and perspective. Methods generally include in-depth interviews and/or focus groups. Less common are participatory action and ethnographic studies.

Philosophically, qualitative inquiry has several conceptual frameworks: ethnography, phenomenology, grounded theory and feminism are a few. These frameworks are steeped in history and assumptions and are beyond the scope of our present discussion.

More commonly, qualitative researchers need to clearly define their methods and can often skirt the issue of conceptual framework, but any author biases need to be clear. The methods need to clarify both how the study was done and what perspective its authors bring to the project, including their culture, profession and gender.

Validity of Qualitative Research

Measures of validity in quantitative research are well developed: the standard of the reproducible experiment and the statistical probability of the "p" value are cornerstones of science. Since qualitative research admits to a subjective worldview and method, validity as defined by scientific method is harder to define – but is critically important. Qualitative inquiry has well-developed measures of reliability and validity.

It exists contentedly within its limitation that its data may not be generalizable. Since the depth of data is the outcome, the deeper the data, the more insight results in understanding the thinking or feeling of one person or group of people.

If one interviews chosen representative subjects of a homogeneous ilk and the interviews render similar themes, one can assume an understanding is developing.

Saturation refers to the process of arriving at no new information while conducting the final several interviews. The assumption is that nothing more will be discovered from interviewing more members of this group of participants. The information gathered may not be generalizable to other groups – but that was not the intention and is indeed the practical trade-off to learning in-depth data.

Triangulation confers validity on one's qualitative results by referring to other sources of collaborating information: other studies, field notes and multiple investigators coding and developing themes. *Member checking* one's results and clearly explaining one's relation to the subjects, type of sampling, and data gathering and analysis build up a measure of trustworthiness.

The bottom line is each method has strength and weaknesses. The question should lend itself to one or the other. One method may also be a better fit for the particular researcher, with more artistic personalities more drawn to qualitative approaches. In a simple world, the question dictates the method and the type of collaborating colleagues the researcher will need to complete the project.

Scientific methods and positivism were an emancipation of sorts. Objective reality was now discoverable by everyman. There was no need for a philosopher-king, or a church-hierarchy to interpret reality. Because it has been such a powerful socio-political and philosophical movement, its dominant effect should not surprise us – nor should it deter us from visiting other assumptions and research methods. If we had to create Jungian mandalas for each of the two traditional research "ways of knowing," one would be the organized face of a clock, the other the mingled face of a pizza. They each have something to contribute and are interpreted in different ways!

Reflexivity

Can your values, acquaintances, political views and biases influence your research work? How are our research question, methodology and results reflections of ourselves?

The concept of reflexivity has a complex sociological and philosophical history dating back to the 1920s. The concept began describing the bidirectional flow of influence between cause and effect. One changes the other in an on-going dialect. A passive anthropologist observing an isolated forest tribe changes their social structure by being there and simply observing. In qualitative research, reflexivity identifies the biases we bring to the table. This style of research has done a reasonable job in admitting the effect of researcher bias while viewing human behavior through a human lens. Bias is acknowledged in the methods section in two ways. Initially, by referencing a particular conceptual framework and secondly, by identifying the profession, perspective and role of the researcher, and the context of the relationship with the participants. We set the stage of the play and the players before the first act begins.

Quantitative research has not traveled long down this pathway. Researchers typically have to acknowledge any conflict of interest – but that is generally limited to a disclosure of the receipt of some financial teaching or research support. The perspective of the quantitative researcher is a product of their social, professional and personal environment. Can that affect their research? If it has an effect on the questions they pose, then it will affect the results they produce. This may explain why guidelines produced primarily by clinicians who deal with only one disease often do not fit well for the generalists expected to apply them. The personal and professional perspective we have is not a limitation. It is a part of the research operation itself. Reflexivity refers to the acknowledgement of one's biases, so that the research can be accurately appreciated.

TEACHING RESEARCH

Most medical schools have critical appraisal courses for assessing journal articles and research reports for accuracy and relevance. Training in research methods is less common, even though research projects are often required of some undergraduate learners and most postgraduate learners. The community-based clinical teacher has a limited role to play, depending on their own facility with research, but collaborating with a student on their project could be educational. Many community preceptors will have graduated after the boom of evidence-based medicine and critical appraisal. These "critical-reading" skills are second nature to most present-generation medical undergraduates. By the time they graduate and are residents, they hone their critical appraisal skills during journal clubs. If the preceptor is behind in this capacity, then set aside some time to be the learner and get your student to "begin class." They will be surprised and pleased, but they will be able to teach you quite a bit. Have them do this during lunch rounds for those colleagues who are similarly afflicted.

If the preceptor is involved in critically appraising the literature on topics affecting their practice, or is developing research projects, involving the student accomplishes two things. It gives you help in getting things started, especially with some of the library/search and article retrieval steps. It also gives you added impetus to eventually complete the project, so that the learner's work does not go for naught.

Even if neither teacher not learner is particularly involved in research, case discussions might include use of landmark papers, the meaning of "p" value, the vast difference between the often-quoted relative risk-reduction versus the more comprehensive absolute-risk reduction value. Outcome measures are also an important concept to demonstrate to learners. The use of composite or surrogate endpoints may not carry the weight of clinical endpoints that are often more relevant to integrating research findings into actual patient care decisions. A robust discussion of absolute and relative-risk reduction, number needed to treat, specificity and sensitivity takes place in Chapter 25, (p. 222).

LITERATURE SEARCHING

Since almost all research projects must start with going to the literature to see what is already documented on your topic, it bears some attention. Doing a quick look for up-to-date articles is an easy first step. "Dr. Google" may even help out with a recent scholarly journal article on the subject. However, a comprehensive literature search will ultimately be required for developing a research project. Searches can be quite frustrating, so keep in mind that many libraries' may do the search for you. Even if someone else completes the search for you, it is worthwhile to know about how searches and databases work.

A preliminary search looking for review articles is a reasonable place to start. A more thorough search may take three or more hours to review abstracts and decide on relevant papers. Articles can often be retrieved online at the time of your search, particularly if you are using a university affiliated library service that has arranged copyright access for its users.

After an initial read of the literature, you will have a better idea of where your research idea fits. Has it been investigated in your patient population? Has it been studied in geographic areas where distance can affect treatment? The literature may also sufficiently broaden the scope of your topic to make it undoable for you. It is important, at this point, to compose the title of your proposed work and write it down. This will help you to focus both cognitively and practically. It will help you avoid being led down any interesting but unproductive avenues offered by a broad search strategy. Having the topic written down gives you a cognitive reference point and something to refer back to when the topic seems to be expanding before your eyes.

Textword or Keyword Searches

If we want to look up references to the exact words we use, then we would want to search for these as "keywords" or "textwords." This search would give us articles which use the specific term in the title or even in the body of the papers. A keyword search is, therefore, good for very specific or exact terms. If, however, you perform a keyword search on a common or general term such as "rural," you will get hundreds of thousands of articles listed; too many to be useful. So use keyword searches for very specific terms only, such as "Cree," one of North America's specific First Nations.

MeSH Terms

The descriptive language we use changes over time. Many library databases were established in the 1950s using the best terms of that time to organize vast numbers of articles. Search terms established in these databases are typically called MeSH, medical subject headings. For example, in Canada, the present politically and socially acceptable term "First Nations" is referenced under the medical subject heading in the MEDLINE database of "Indians, North American." The MeSH term and the language we currently use are quite different. The librarians anticipated this problem and have programmed some search engines to do the translation for us – without us knowing it.

Typically, we would conduct a MeSH search if performing a comprehensive search. This strategy will give us the benefit of having the search engine deliver a composite of results which includes the terms we use, as well different ones by other researchers who have used slightly different entry terms. The joy of it is that you do not need to know the specific MeSH term to enter; the program will often do it for you. It is useful to know this distinction between MeSH searches and keyword searches as background information before we discuss search engines and databases.

PubMed and MEDLINE are very similar databases for medical information. The differences lie in their search strategies default settings: one looks for keywords, the other for MeSH terms (*see* Figure 20.3).

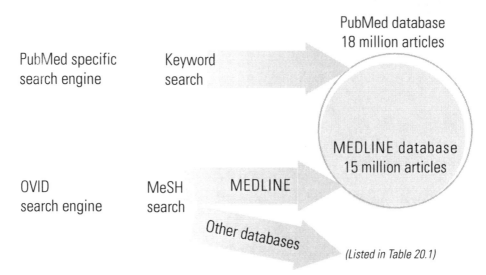

Figure 20.3 Default Settings of Common Search Engines

PubMed database searches are performed through its own search engine (called Entrez) which looks for keywords. MEDLINE search done through the common engine called OVID, performs MeSH searches. As we have seen, these can give diverse results. Either search engine can be asked to search in either keyword or MeSH terms, but their default strategy is as stated. If you prefer the PubMed interface, you can ask it to perform a MeSH search and you will then achieve almost identical results to an OVID-MEDLINE search. The PubMed database uses its own search engine. On the other hand, the OVID search engine can access many databases. We have listed some of them below.

Table 20.1 Databases Searchable by OVID

MEDLINE	1950	15 million articles > 5000 medical journals
EMBASE	1974	18 million articles; biomedical and pharmaceutical: includes European literature
CINAHL	1982	Cumulative index to nursing and allied health literature
HealthSTAR	1975	MEDLINE plus hospital, government, technical reports
PSYCHINFO	1872	Psychology; was PsycLIT

EMB Reviews	1948	Included Cochrane, American College of Physicians (ACP) Journal Club
NATIVE HEALTH DATABASE	1966	North American Aboriginal documents surveys
AMED	1985	Allied and complementary: OT, PT, podiatry, palliative care, complementary medicine

After this initial work has been done, it is time to follow the remaining "commandments." Collaborate, choose a methodology and scope of project and keep moving forward, following a journal writing template to control the length and organization of the work.

SUMMARY

However deeply one plans to delve into research in one's practice, it is always healthy to maintain a healthy sense of curiosity and even skepticism about what medical research brings us. The language is often changing and this can be very intimidating to most clinicians. This is an unfortunate consequence of the increasingly complex language of research. There is only so much time and energy we can apply to research activities, if our main focus is our clinical practice. As distributed education evolves, the academic needs of community-based clinical teachers should become recognized and supported, and this includes research. Then protected time and access to experienced statisticians, mentors and researchers may need to be available. By the same token, community clinical educators who choose to focus just on their practice and teaching responsibilities can leave research to others if they choose.

FURTHER READING

Barbour R. Checklists for improving rigour in qualitative research: a case of the tail wagging the dog? *BMJ*. 2001; **322**: 1115. doi:10.1136/bmj.322.7294.1115

Feldman A, Force T, Whellan D, *et al.* Advancing the research mission in an academic department: the creation of a center for translational medicine. Available at: www. CTSjournal.com. DOI: 10.1111/j.1752-8062.2010.00206.x (accessed August 9, 2011)

Kelly L. Developing a rural research project. *CJRM*. 2008; **13**(4): 194–6.

Kelly L, St Pierre-Hansen N. So many databases, such little clarity. *Can Fam Phys*. 2008; **54**: 1572–3; e1–5.

Mays N, Pope C. Assessing quality in qualitative research. *BMJ*. 2000; **320**(7226): 50–2.

Nagy Hesse-Biber S, Leavy P. *The Practice of Qualitative Research*. Thousand Oaks, CA: Sage Publications; 2006.

21

Professional Development

Ruth Wilson, Jeff Sloan and Len Kelly

Career development sits in balance with the rest of one's life: personal and family growth. The balance is dynamic and can assume different directions during various phases of one's personal and professional life. Development of non-work-related pastimes is likely one of the more neglected aspects of a healthy career in medicine. An obsessive career which brings praise, but little peace, will not serve us well. There is a need for balance.

Medical vocations often have choices for which we feel unprepared: choosing a residency program, a work location, a style, type or amount of work. These are all hallmark decisions we make along the way. Learning to say "no" to increased workloads is a key survival skill. That may mean turning down career options when they arise. We might be better prepared if we understood some of the options in professional development, so that we might chart our course, flexible as it might need to be.

Overwork is a vocational liability but it may not need to be the best route to professional advancement.

Lastly, the clinical teacher's personality must be a good fit for on-going career choices, whether they are maintaining their status quo or a changing focus. Focusing one's career on developing specific knowledge of one area of medicine may not sit well with a generalist and vice versa.

FURTHER TRAINING
Additional Clinical Training
One of the first questions a graduate clinician faces is whether to do further training before leaving the "hallowed halls" and safety of residency. Extra skillsets both open doors and close them. A family physician that does extra training in anesthesia will be limited to communities which: appreciate GP/anesthesia training, have vacancies and have a surgical program. Some extra skills such as obstetrics may be best practiced in a supportive group practice. Knowing where you will practice can be very helpful, but is not always possible.

Continuing on as a learner has a good comfort level as long as the skill will fit well into future plans and practice locations.

Another strategy is to settle into one's practice and see what the community needs are, how onerous they might be on the practitioner to provide, and what access and funding exists for "re-entry" positions. In this scenario, the clinician can tailor their learning to fit well with community needs. The drawback is that the clinician will often suffer financially and need to spend time away from family to acquire these skills.

POST GRADUATE DEGREES

A Master's degree or research fellowship training are increasingly becoming accessible by distant education venues. While they take longer than full-time studies (i.e. 2–5 years for a Master's degree) they can be done part-time from one's home community. The questions arise: "What do I want to learn" and "Why?"

These degrees are a lot of work but can break down many intellectual barriers. A rural physician may, in time, feel like a second or poor cousin to those closer to university centers. Delving into topics related to teaching or research by becoming a mature student may address that. While these degrees may be done concurrently or immediately following clinical training, they may have a better fit for many of us after our practice is established. Then the practicalities of work and family life are established (though never fixed). At this 5–10-year mark, one can choose which degree might best satisfy one's curiosity. The key element needed for undertaking additional learning is to protect time. Keep in mind that colleagues who undertake employment at a university academic clinical center will often have 1–2 days per week of protected time for several years to accomplish an advanced degree. You need to be able to protect time in other ways in order to invest in changes to your career.

ACADEMIC PROMOTION

Lecturer, assistant, associate and then, full professor. These historically steeped stages of academic advancement are often an awkward fit for clinical teachers. In the past, they signified one's achievements and one's pay scale. Today, most clinical teachers typically generate their income through patient care duties and these titles are essentially honorary.

You may not be interested in academic promotion, and may find the rewards of teaching are intrinsic. However, if you do wish to be promoted, here are some suggestions.

➤ *Document:* A great deal of the work you do in teaching is useful in preparing a teaching dossier to support your application. Every time you give a talk, teach a student, make a presentation at a meeting or chair a committee, keep a copy in a file (electronic or otherwise) so that, when the time comes, you can appropriately collate the evidence to support your application.

➤ *Learn the rules:* Each university has a slightly different set of rules for promotion. Some universities have a track for promoting clinician teachers; others do not. In some universities, creative activities such as the radio broadcast you have been doing for years in aid of health promotion in your community "count"– but they will not in others.

➤ *Find a mentor:* If you are interested in pursuing academic promotion, it is useful to have a mentor who has been through the process. Your department head might fill this role for you; he or she has an interest in making sure that faculty members are promoted appropriately.

➤ *Don't be shy:* Putting forward an application for promotion involves a fair amount of self-promotion and putting together a portfolio to show the scholarly work you have done. This does not come naturally to many of us, but is a requirement for advancement in academia.

➤ *Be scholarly:* The essence of what is required for academic promotion is scholarly work. Scholarly work entails critical reflection about the work you do, creation of new knowledge, and dissemination of your ideas through publication or presentations. The hard currency of academia is publication. There are many resources to help you with publication of your thoughts and findings. Your university department and your professional associations are good places to start.

GEOGRAPHIC FULL-TIME STATUS

A century ago, medical schools relied on physicians with private practices who would teach on the public wards of hospitals for their faculty. A system pioneered by Johns Hopkins brought the teaching physician into the realm of the faculty medicine. There, geographic full-time (GFT) physicians made all of their patients available for teaching, and devoted their full professional effort to the work of the faculty.

In Canadian medical faculties this GFT concept, with some changes, still applies. GFT physicians are devoting all their efforts to teaching and research within the university, and do not have private non-teaching practices. In many Canadian faculties, GFT physicians received a salary (so-called "hard" dollars) in recognition of their contributions, although the bulk of their income is likely still made up of clinical earnings. Some universities appoint GFT faculty but do not pay any salary to them.

There are a couple of twists on the GFT designation – each of the letters in the acronym may not mean exactly what it says. It is possible to be a part-time GFT: the idea is that even though one is working part-time, one is devoting one's full professional effort to the institution. This designation can be labeled as "GFT with reduced responsibility." The Geographic part of the designation is also now more loosely interpreted, and it is not uncommon for faculties to appoint GFT faculty who do not live in the same city as the university – part of the push for distributed medical education.

RANK AND TENURE

Initial faculty appointments are generally made at the level of instructor or lecturer. Usually these appointments would be for faculty members who work in a private practice and do some teaching. There would be no expectation of scholarly work for these individuals. Most GFT faculty would be appointed at the level of assistant professor. It would be expected that such appointees would begin to do scholarly work as well as teaching. After seven years as an assistant professor, some faculties offer the chance to apply for promotion to associate professor. An individual applying would be expected to have a strong teaching dossier, evidence of a research program, and a track record of publications, some of which would be as a first author.

In some faculties, application for tenure may be made at the time of application for promotion to associate professor. Tenure implies that a faculty member may only be dismissed for cause, or for reasons of financial exigency on the part of the institution. Tenure has been seen as a key part of academic freedom, since the university would not be able to dismiss a professor for holding or promulgating an unpopular opinion. Tenure has also been seen as important for providing financial stability to the professoriate, enabling them to concentrate on scholarly work.

Tenure has not been as important for medical faculties, as physicians have the opportunity to pursue their profession outside the academy. Some major faculties do not offer tenure. When it is offered, it is generally awarded for individuals meeting the requirements for associate professor.

Promotion to professor (also called "full professor") is not based on any particular time in the academy. Generally, the individual seeking recognition at this level will need national or international recognition of their teaching or scholarly work, including publications, teaching awards and grants.

Administrative service, such as being a program director, is not generally considered in the academic promotion process.

TOWN AND GOWN

There are commonly attitudes from community-based physicians toward those in the ivory tower of academia. Much of it is attitudinal. Being outside the four walls of academic centers leaves one at a perceived disadvantage: no subsidized offices or administrative support and perhaps even better access to specialized services for one's patients. These differences may, in fact, not exist and many primary care physicians in academic centers make less income than their community-based neighbors. Nonetheless, the gap exists and programs need to make an effort to be inclusive to community-based educators, as they are the backbone of the increasingly distributed education reality. They will often be outside the "corporate culture and speak" which develops in most institutions and programs. One community-based preceptor who attended an academic teaching center event recounted:

> "I remember volunteering for a role-play exercise. I didn't do a particularly good job at it and didn't receive much support or encouragement from any of my colleagues. It left me feeling inadequate. It seemed that most of the other attendees were from academic centers and were more or less involved in full-time teaching. It was not a good experience for me and I probably avoided further events of this kind for some years afterwards. I was very intimidated by the academics, even though many of them probably had less teaching experience than me.
>
> To this day, I don't find full time GFT family medicine teachers to be very supportive of the community preceptors — there seems to be a bit of an ivory tower syndrome. For our part, the community preceptors have a bit of smugness to our learning environment where learners are exposed to 'real medicine'."

Faculty development events designed to include community preceptors need to be "accessible, fun, relevant and involve spouses." This community-based clinical educator went on to say that:

> "The idea of attending faculty development sessions for community physicians is analogous to attending sessions on psychiatry and counseling: the topics are 'soft' and not as attractive as learning life-saving skills like rapid sequence induction or chest tube insertion. I do sense a trend toward acceptance of faculty development as necessary, particularly by younger preceptors and perhaps that is where the energy should be focused."

Community-based clinical teachers may, therefore, have a strained relationship with many academic programs. This cultural divide is somewhat inevitable but needs constant attention. Programs need to do some "reaching out" and ensure community physicians feel welcome and supported.

PROFESSIONAL DEVELOPMENT OUTSIDE OF ACADEMIA

Many community organizations need participation from professionals and would love to see a physician on their Board or attending their meetings or sporting events. Giving time and energy to a cause close to one's heart will develop vital community relations and friendships outside of the office.

Other areas that benefit from physician expertise include medical colleges and administrative organizations. These are primarily constituted by physician members. Medico-legal and policy development work are important aspects of the profession. These contributions sometimes lead to paid part- or full-time employment opportunities to the right physician-member. These time and energy contributions often generate long-standing collegial and personal relations that can span a lifetime.

Many physicians can remain competent in several parallel "careers." I know of a retired radiologist who has authored several dozen books and an active urban emergency physician who regularly gives classical music concerts!

SUMMARY

Many of us do not proactively charter a career path, but family, health and educational issues sometimes require a clinician to relocate or redirect their career. Professional contacts and career development come in useful at these times, as well as their intrinsic value. When active clinical work is limited by age or interest, other venues for self-actualization will be needed. Retirement planning inhabits one of the latter stages of professional development and will need to be acknowledged sooner or later!

FURTHER READING

Kaplan P. *Lifting a Ton of Feathers*. Toronto, Ontario, Canada: University of Toronto Press; 1994.

Website
www.aamc.org/members/gfa/gfa_resurces/164742/aps_artucles_collection.html (accessed August 9, 2011)

22

Teaching Professionalism

James Goertzen

Professionalism is largely contextual and best understood as a series of behaviors within a clinical setting, rather than a series of personal character traits or attributes. The challenge for preceptors is to translate and make the concepts of professionalism relevant within clinical practice. It is important to link the principles of professionalism to physicians' relationships with individual patients and families; relationships with other physicians, professional colleagues and healthcare professional team members; relationships with communities and larger society; and relationship with self. This transforms abstract and theoretical knowledge to relevant professional behaviors essential to the practice of medicine. The basic principles of physician professionalism include: accountability, altruism, competence, duty, honor, integrity respect, responsibility and self-regulation.

Professionalism is a core competency essential for medical students, residents and practicing physicians. The development of medical professionalism by our learners is a process that begins on the first day of medical school and continues throughout undergraduate and postgraduate training. The acquisition of professionalism follows a parallel process to the attainment of clinical competence within medical education. Community-based physicians have critical roles in assisting the development of professionalism by learners throughout the educational continuum. We may be involved in some of the undergraduate educational activities that include communication and interview skills or medical ethics. But our central role as preceptors is within a community setting where we will have an individual relationship with a learner over a block of time with multiple clinically based experiences and conversations. These clinical encounters can provide opportunities to teach, role-model and refine the essence of professionalism. Hopefully, upon residency completion, a physician emerges with well-established professional behaviors along with the self-reflection skills necessary to refine these behaviors in response to the challenges of every changing patient and societal expectations.

When learners arrive in our community practice, they will have had some curriculum devoted to the cognitive aspects of professionalism and we can expect a foundation of confidentiality, respect, responsibility and integrity. During the orientation phase of the clinical placement, common principles to cover include commitment to clinic and hospital schedules, along with responsibilities in these settings. The learner may be responsible for assessing hospital patients and composing clinical notes prior to rounding with the preceptor to foster learner-independence and provide opportunities for feedback on clinical and professional competence. Since, within a family medicine clinical context, learners of all levels will often assess patients independently prior to review with their preceptor, clarifications around learner and preceptor professional responsibilities with this model of clinical and educational care are essential. Upon review of the clinical encounter, a professional standard the learner would be expected to meet would include being honest about their clinical comfort, competence and inadvertent omissions. For the preceptor, an acceptable professional standard would include a willingness to accept questions and challenges to their preferred clinical approaches, along with building in time in the weekly schedule for more in-depth discussion or reflection when necessary.

The majority of a learner's professional development will occur within the clinical setting. This will include role-modeling by their preceptor and observation by the learner. In addition other physicians and healthcare professionals will also influence a learner through their actions and interactions. Role-modeling will include both positive and negative attributes. Thus, reflection by the learner is essential as they incorporate observed professional behaviors. A learner's professional behaviors will be further crystallized by reinforcement and feedback from their preceptor, other healthcare professionals and patients.

The challenge for preceptors when teaching professionalism is to move from seemingly haphazard clinical encounters to purposeful clinical experiences which can be used to observe the learner's professional behaviors, provide opportunities for clinically related conversations to encourage learner reflection, and form the basis for specific feedback related to observed behaviors. Purposeful clinical encounters can be chosen because of their specific content or context, such as learner involvement with patients of different ethnic backgrounds, care of dying patients or those with a chronic disease with limited treatment options, communicating bad or unexpected news, or review of DNR status. In addition, involving learners in common clinical encounters such as a patient with a common cold can be purposeful when the encounter is used as a spring-board for discussion of potential patient–physician conflict, around the prescribing of antibiotics, request for diagnostic tests, or negotiating the length of work absence. Key to the content-rich or seemingly mundane clinical encounter is the dialogue that follows with preceptor and learner where conversation and reflection are encouraged and positive professional behaviors are recognized and reinforced. The dialogue takes into consideration the stage of the learner's training along with their emotional and professional maturity. Key to the discussion is a confidential and safe educational environment where honesty, disclosure and reflection are valued.

Lapses in professional behavior by our learners are common and to be expected (*see* Table 22.1). It is through the experience of learning within a supervised clinical setting that the principles of professionalism can be truly integrated. Common professional lapses by medical students include inappropriate or miscommunication with patients and other healthcare professionals, derogatory comments about patients or other healthcare professionals, the objectification of patients and not addressing program or patient expectations. A lapse in professional behavior by a medical student or resident can be transformed into a critical teaching and learning scenario where we can have a collegial conversation with our learner, encouraging reflection and assimilation of appropriate professional behaviors. Ample opportunity should initially be given to the learner to explain the clinical context and rationale for their seemingly unprofessional behavior. In many clinical encounters, there may be competition between two or more seemingly divergent professional or personal values. Thus, the context is central for the learner as they resolve possible conflicting values that are then expressed through their specific behavior. If a preceptor assumes that, for each clinical situation, there is one right answer in terms of professionalism, meaningful dialogue will be limited, with the learner becoming defensive and minimizing the possibility of meaningful reflection. It is important for the preceptor to understand the process used by the learner to arrive at their expressed professional behaviour, in order to develop effective educational interventions that are collegial and learner-specific when professional missteps are made.

Lapses of professional behavior occur on a continuum. The majority will involve a conversation where the preceptor has a full understanding of the

Table 22.1 Lapses in Professionalism

➤ Some minor lapses in professionalism are common
➤ Lapses occur along a continuum of severity, with implications for patient and learner outcomes
➤ Minor lapses include: inappropriate corridor conversations, criticism of colleagues, late attendance
➤ More serious lapses include: inattentiveness to patient care, not communicating significant results to preceptor, derogatory comments about patients or healthcare professionals, lying
➤ Most serious lapses include: dating a patient, inappropriate prescribing

context, along with process the learner used. Following learner reflection, the lapse can be acknowledged and learner commitment for behavioral change explored. Observation and monitoring by the preceptor, along with providing additional clinical encounters to address the professionalism lapse with specific feedback, and appropriate reinforcement for the learner may suffice. Preceptors should retain brief notes on the lapse, for incorporation into the mid-term or final rotation evaluation.

If lapses reoccur or are of a more serious nature, a staged response is appropriate. The format of a collegial conversation with clarification of context, learner process, learner reflection and planning of future learning activities should still be followed, much as we do with the difficult learner. Learners must be notified of any consequences of not improving their professional behavior, and the learner's program director may need to be notified. Involving the learner's educational program provides additional resources and support to both the preceptor and learner. In addition, the program director can ensure that the preceptor is following the process required for addressing recurrent or serious unprofessional behavior.

It is critical that preceptors address lapses of professionalism by learners during their medical training, since there is evidence that medical student unprofessional behavior is associated with disciplinary action by licensing bodies, following graduation. Students with the strongest association were described as irresponsible (unreliable attendance at clinics and not following up on activities related to patient care) and having a diminished capacity to improve (failure to accept constructive criticism, argumentativeness and display of poor attitude).

SUMMARY

Professionalism is a core competency during undergraduate and postgraduate training. Preceptors have a central role in modeling and teaching professionalism throughout clinical rotations. Professional lapses by our learners are to be expected and are an invitation for a collegial conversation to better understand the context of the specific clinical encounter and acknowledge potential conflict between competing professional and personal values for the learner. Linking the conversation with an opportunity for learner reflection provides the framework for the development of future learning activities linked to preceptor observation and specific feedback. This results in a learner who will more likely incorporate the principles of professionalism, as part of independent practice. along with having the reflective skills to adjust and address changing patient and societal expectations.

FURTHER READING

Hafferty F. Professionalism – the next wave. *NEMJ*. 2006; **355**: 2151–2.

Papadakis M, Hodgson C, Teherani A, *et al*. Unprofessional behaviour in medical school is associated with subsequent disciplinary action by a state medical board. *Acad Med*. 2004; **79**: 244–9.

Stern D, Papadakis M. The developing physician – becoming a professional. *NEMJ*. 2006; **355**: 1794–9.

Van Mook W, De Grave W, Gorter S, *et al*. Intensive care medicine trainees' perception of professionalism: a qualitative study. *Anesth Int Care*. 2011; **39**(1): 107–15.

23

Relationships and Boundaries

Leslie Rourke and James Rourke

"It is Sunday morning and you, your spouse, and children are all packed and about to leave for a day at the beach about an hour's drive away. Everyone has been looking forward to this all week. You are not on call. The telephone rings. It is a friend you regularly golf with, who is also your patient. He says he has severe abdominal pain, and asks if you can come to see him at his home."

One of the joys of community practice is the opportunity to know our patients beyond the doctor–patient relationship. Our patients may be neighbors, colleagues, staff, friends, or the bank manager. Knowing patients in roles other than the straight forward doctor–patient relationship adds richness and connectedness to our work. However, it can also add significant challenge and stress, altering both the doctor–patient relationship and the personal relationship.

Rural physicians have many such "special" patients – those with whom they have multi-dimensional (multi-faceted) relationships. However, this is not unique to rural practice. Complex relationships with patients can, and do, occur for all physicians in any sized community and within any specialty. The subspecialist in a large center who sees all cases from the region will likely need to treat colleagues and friends. The radiologist may well face the situation of having to tell a friend that her mammogram is strongly suspicious of breast cancer. Beyond the relationship complexities faced by the physician, family members of a physician may face challenges when seeking medical care from the physician's colleagues.

Relationship issues also tend to become more complex over the course of one's career. Clinical expertise is expected to increase with experience, with the result that the diagnosis and management become more accustomed over time. In contrast, social interconnectedness becomes wider and deeper over time, with the result that the challenges of a dual- (or triple-) faceted relationship become more complex. What is the solution when the best candidate for an office receptionist position is a patient? Or when there is pressure to hire a colleague's family member?

Finally, relationship and boundary issues are not as readily learned from medical textbooks as are clinical scenarios, differential diagnoses or drugs of choice. Relationship issues in conventional medical school teaching have tended to be ignored, downplayed or marginalized. However, community physicians live with the reality of complex and multi-dimensional doctor–patient relationships. The challenges of such relationships can cause significant stress and impact career satisfaction.

We will outline challenges with, and strategies for, the successful negotiation of complex and multi-dimensional doctor–patient relationships. Our intent is to provide clinical teachers with the skillset to help learners develop an awareness of relationship and boundary issues.

BOUNDARIES AND ETHICAL DECISION-MAKING PRINCIPLES

By "boundary" we mean the accepted social, psychological and physical space between people. Boundaries are explicitly and implicitly defined by culture, jurisprudence and ethics. The appropriateness of any given boundary is also influenced by individual, personal, environmental and professional factors.

Types of boundaries that are important to the doctor–patient relationship include: clothing limitations, form of address, gifts, doctor self-disclosure and social media networking (social boundaries); touch and time and place of access (physical boundaries).

It is particularly important for learners to be aware of boundary issues. Medical students and residents undergo multiple changes in role and status relative to other learners and to patients as they move through the learning stages from pre-clerkship to clerkship to professional. With each change in role and status, the boundaries between the learner and patients change, both in quality and in significance. Decision-making also becomes increasingly the onus of responsibility of the learner; situations can arise suddenly with the need for immediate decision-making. It is essential for the emerging professional to have insight into potential ethical dilemmas related to boundary issues before an ethical dilemma requiring fast decision-making is required.

An understanding of ethical decision-making principles helps in difficult boundary issues. When boundaries are an issue, ask:

➤ Is there a conflict of interest?
➤ Do relations of power come into play?
➤ Is the standard of care provided being lessened because of the blurred boundaries?

CONFLICTS OF INTEREST

A conflict of interest occurs when one's judgment regarding a primary interest may be unduly influenced by a secondary interest. For example, when a member of a physician's office staff becomes ill, there may be a conflict of interest if that staff member is also a patient of the physician. In the role of physician, it is in the best interests of the patient to have the staff member sent home to recuperate; in the role of office manager, it is in the best interests of the functioning of the office to have the staff member remain at work despite being ill. It is not unethical to *be in* a conflict of interest. It is unethical to allow a secondary interest to take precedence over what has been established as the primary interest. In this example, not suggesting time off work for the staff member if it was warranted, due to the effect on the office, would be an unethical outcome *if* it has been determined that the primary relationship is that of doctor and patient.

POWER DIFFERENTIALS

It is important that learners understand the power differential in the doctor–patient relationship (*see* Figure 23.1). The doctor is a powerful authority figure who not only operates as gatekeeper to investigations, medications and other therapeutic modalities, but also validates the patient's sick role to society (e.g. granting time off work). Note that the healthcare team itself is comprised of members with varying roles, responsibilities and statuses; if not sensitively managed, power differentials can have a negative impact on team functioning. Similarly, there is a power differential between the teacher and the learner. These power differentials will be further discussed in the section entitled "Relationship and boundary issues and learners."

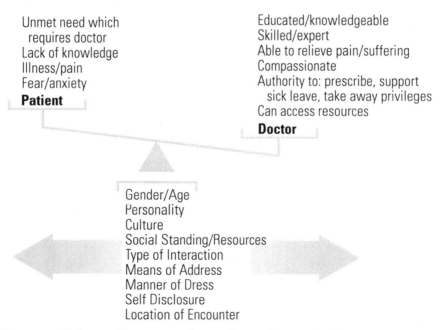

Unmet need which
  requires doctor
Lack of knowledge
Illness/pain
Fear/anxiety
Patient

Educated/knowledgeable
Skilled/expert
Able to relieve pain/suffering
Compassionate
Authority to: prescribe, support
  sick leave, take away privileges
Can access resources
Doctor

Gender/Age
Personality
Culture
Social Standing/Resources
Type of Interaction
Means of Address
Manner of Dress
Self Disclosure
Location of Encounter

Figure 23.1 Balance of Power in the Doctor–Patient Relationship. [Adapted from Dunn]

STANDARD OF CARE

Standard of care can be affected when the doctor–patient relationship is complicated by boundary issues. Omission of care, assumptions, breaches of confidentiality and loss of objectivity resulting in under- or over-investigation or treatment can all affect standard of care in these cases. (*See* the section later in this chapter entitled *Risks related to medical care for "special patients"* for examples and alternatives for medical care in these situations).

BOUNDARY VIOLATIONS

A boundary violation can occur in three ways: 1 there is a blurring of the difference between personal and professional roles; 2 there is a role-reversal where the physician's needs take precedence over the patient's needs; or 3 the behavioral rules expected of people in a given role are transgressed. Boundary violations are more likely to occur with high-risk patients, high-risk situations and high-risk doctors.

High-risk Patients

Not surprisingly, patients at high-risk for boundary violations with physicians are those with their own boundary issues. Those patients at highest risk are victims of abuse or people with borderline personality disorder. Patients with chronic neediness, dependence or prior relationship problems are at moderate risk. Even low-risk patients with no prior boundary problems can become at risk at times of stress.

"Special patients" – those with multi-dimensional relationships with the physician – such as personal friends, are also at risk for boundary violations due to their special access to and relationship with the physician.

High-risk Situations

Examples of high-risk situations include taking a sexual history, conducting a physical examination, providing psychotherapy and providing care in an unusual setting (time or place). Professionalism during patient encounters, including respect and putting the patient's needs foremost, helps to protect against boundary violations and can be discussed and modelled for the learner. (*see* Table 23.1).

High-risk Physicians

Physicians at high-risk for boundary violations include those who have significant physical, emotional or sexual problems or unresolved needs; are naive or have a particular blind spot; have an impulse control problem; or are paternalistic, grandiose, authoritarian or entitled.

Being an expert in medical knowledge does not exempt one from physical, mental, emotional or social problems. Physicians are humans with personality

Table 23.1 Professionalism During Patient Encounters. (Adapted from *Violence Issues for Health Care Educators and Providers*, Graham A, Hamberger LK and Burge SK, 1997, with permission of Haworth Press/Taylor and Francis Books.)

> ➤ Know yourself, your boundaries and your biases. Examine your values and use of language
> ➤ Know your patients and respect their boundaries
> ➤ Learn to be technically good at what you do
> ➤ Admit when something is beyond your area of expertise and consult if appropriate
> ➤ Before doing an examination or procedure, explain and ask permission
> ➤ For breast, pelvic, rectal or GU exams, consider/offer or obtain third party presence.
> ➤ Do not do a sexual history during this exam
> ➤ Respect privacy with undressing and draping
> ➤ Give the patient some control during the physical examination. Explain what you are doing
> ➤ If something hurts, stop. Correct the situation and ask permission to proceed

traits and past experiences which influence the way of approaching relationships, patterns of dealing with stress and so on. Any physician can be at risk of a boundary violation – hence the importance of recognizing" red flags" for boundary violations and sharing these with our learners (*see* Table 23.2). The College of Physicians and Surgeons of Ontario Canada has published a self-assessment tool of 27 questions to raise awareness of, encourage self-reflection on, and promote open discussion regarding boundary issues, which can also serve as an excellent teaching tool with learners (*see* end of chapter Further Reading). Equally important is physician self-care of emotional health and strategies for handling stress.

Table 23.2 Recognizing Red Flags for Boundary Violations. (Adapted from *Violence Issues for Health Care Educators and Providers*, Graham A, Hamberger LK and Burge SK, 1997, with permission of Haworth Press/Taylor and Francis Books.)

> ➤ Making exceptions: "I don't usually do this"
> ➤ Seeking social contact with patients or doing therapy during social situations
> ➤ Responding to pressure from the patient to disclose personal information
> ➤ Confiding with patients about our personal/marital problems
> ➤ Daydreaming about/longing for the patient
> ➤ Setting up after-hours appointments
> ➤ Driving the patient home
> ➤ Accepting inappropriate gifts from the patient
> ➤ Wanting to "rescue" the patient
> ➤ Trying to impress the patient with our personal achievements or our "specialness"
> ➤ Being gratified by a sense of power when a patient's activity is controlled through our advice, medication or behavioral restraint

Physician professional associations have codes of ethics to guide physicians, and physician licensing bodies have policies regarding misconduct involving boundary violations. When in doubt about a potential boundary violation, always seek advice. Model advice-seeking for learners.

RISKS RELATED TO MEDICAL CARE FOR "SPECIAL" PATIENTS

There are several risks related to the standard of medical care when caring for "special" patients, those patients with multi-dimensional relationships with the physician.

Omission can occur by either patient or physician. For example, a patient may be less comfortable in disclosing the risk of sexually transmitted disease to a physician whose spouse is a close friend of the patient's spouse. The physician may omit personal questions from the history of the patient who is also the physician's child's schoolteacher.

Breaches in confidentiality are a risk when the patient is known to the physician or their family in other roles. One of us (LR) recalls a patient refusing to continue therapy with the local psychiatrist who had greeted the patient by name in the grocery store.

Assumptions can be made by patients who expect the physician to recall aspects of their medical history or family history that would have been learned in a setting other than the clinic.

Loss of objectivity can occur with close friends as patients and can result in either under- or over-investigation or treatment. Emergency situations and terminal illnesses can be particularly stressful and lead to loss of objectivity.

Blurred boundaries are a particular risk as "special" patients often have more access to the physician outside of usual work hours and locations.

Alternatives for Medical Care for "Special" Patients

Alternatives for medical care can be conceptualized into four broad types:

1 The physician does not treat friends

A simple way to avoid boundary violations is for a physician to not enter into a doctor–patient relationship with friends. This strategy is deceptively simple but in practice increasingly difficult. Over time, it becomes virtually impossible in a rural area where local physicians provide on-call coverage for all colleagues' practices. Does the physician opt for very few patients or very few friends?

There are times, however, when a physician should avoid treating the friend (assuming it is not an emergency situation where there is no other option). LaPuma and Priest's classic article *"Is there a doctor in the house? An analysis of the practice of physicians treating their own families"* outlines questions to consider in treating family members. Four of these questions can also apply to these "special" patients:

1   Am I too close to probe my friend's intimate history and physical being?
2   Can I cope with bearing bad news if need be?
3   Can I be objective enough to not give too much, too little, or inappropriate care?
4   Will my friend comply with my medical care as well as he or she would with the care of a physician who was not a friend?

2 The physician treats friends in a more limited way than usual patients

This requires setting tighter boundaries around the doctor–patient relationship than exist with usual patients. One example of a method of tightening boundaries and limiting care is to refer friends who are patients to other physicians for reproductive or psychological problems, but continuing to care for them for non-sensitive issues. Patients or physicians can initiate the limitation of scope of practice depending on their comfort level.

3 The physician treats friends in a more available way than usual patients

A contrasting approach is to loosen the boundaries around the doctor–patient relationship. This strategy is a practical one that results from the patient having greater access to the physician outside of the clinical setting; this loosening of the usual boundaries around the time and place for a medical encounter may also be the result of the "give and take" of friendship favors. The strategy of being more available to patients who are also friends is a common scenario and often exists by "default" as a result of insufficient reflection on the ethical implications of boundary violations. In some instances, the loosening of boundaries around the doctor–patient relationship may be non-problematic, but in most instances, such availability has risks. It may open the door for manipulation of the patient by the doctor or of the doctor by the patient; more significantly, it may lead to a lessening of the standard of care through the risks (omission, assumptions…) outlined above.

4 The physician attempts to treat all patients equitably, whether or not they are also friends

In many instances, it is best to try to treat "special" patients the same as usual patients: seeing them in the clinic situation where a more thorough history and physical exam can result in a more accurate diagnosis and appropriate management. This strategy, more so than the three listed above, may negatively affect the friendship if looser boundaries are expected by the patient as a benefit of the friendship. This type of conflict of interest is best managed by discussion with the friend prior to entering into the doctor–patient relationship (or, conversely, discussion with the patient prior to entering into a friendship). It should also be explicitly reviewed when circumstances of either the professional or personal relationship change.

This approach does not apply to romantic relationships with patients, which are strictly forbidden and are clearly outlined in ethical codes of conduct by professional organizations. Key messages relating to boundary issues are found in Table 23.3.

Table 23.3 Key Messages Relating to Relationships and Boundaries

➤ Be aware of your own unique vulnerabilities
➤ Practice self-care
➤ Be proactive: set guidelines for boundaries
➤ Be conscious of high-risk patients/situations
➤ Be aware when you are tempted to deviate from your usual care
➤ Think of the ethical issues involved
➤ Listen to your gut: recognize that "Oh-oh" feeling
➤ Seek advice

RELATIONSHIP ISSUES FOR THE PHYSICIAN'S SPOUSE AND FAMILY

There are both benefits and challenges to being the spouse and family of a physician. One of the benefits is that medicine is a profession in demand. Physicians rarely have problems with job or financial security. Also, the role of physician (as with healers in most cultures) engenders respect which can extend to the doctor's family. Finally, the physician's spouse and family have a special place when they themselves become patients, sometimes because of (unjust) better access to the medical system, but always because of better access to the privileged "insider" knowledge of the medical community.

These benefits can also present challenges. Medicine is a profession in demand – and it is also a demanding profession, with not only long hours but unpredictable interruptions and intrusions into family life. The physician's spouse cannot only be a "functional single parent" but, in community medicine, can also have the unenviable role of gatekeeper between the doctor and community.

The respect for and high expectations of the physician has likened living with a physician to "living with God." Some physicians also experience the "Titanic syndrome," in which they deny their own vulnerabilities. In contrast, others who have a need to discuss their feelings in difficult patient encounters are in conflict with the need for patient confidentiality. Physician's spouses in this situation may learn confidential medical information about their own friends. In order to remain objective with their patients' heartaches, physicians may learn to be emotionally distant, which can spill over to their personal relationships as well. The perception of spouse and family that they are less important than patients, results in guilt and anger.

Moreover, the physician's spouse and family are *de facto* "special" patients, with all the associated complexities discussed earlier.

RELATIONSHIP AND BOUNDARY ISSUES AND LEARNERS

It is important to understand that the power differential, which exists in the doctor–patient relationship, also exists in the teacher–learner relationship. It is the duty of clinical supervisors to be aware of, and maintain, an acceptable educational and clinical hierarchical relationship between the professional physician and the learner. Learners, too, need to understand and respect the hierarchical nature of the relationship with their clinical supervisor. That is, discussions of boundary maintenance with learners should make explicit the nature of the supervisor–learner relationship as well as the nature of the doctor–patient boundaries that affect all medical staff and their patients.

Learners are professional colleagues of their preceptor. While there may often be a friendliness arising from shared clinical care, and sometimes shared family meals, *we need not be friends to all of our learners.* In fact, this is one of the first boundary issues we must work out with our learners, that the teacher–learner relationship is a professional one.

Our learners will be in professional relationships – and sometimes also in multi-faceted or complex relationships – with our office staff, patients, colleagues, community and us. The boundaries will need to be discussed and made explicit at times, and may need to be emphasized for certain learners or specific contexts.

Professional Conduct

Learners are obliged to appear and act professionally. This may seem commonsensical, but the need to be explicit to learners about professional conduct becomes painfully obvious when professional conduct is not upheld. The clinical teacher may feel embarrassed to point out such a basic and assumed requirement to a learner; it may be necessary to enlist the help or opinion of an office manager or colleague if the situation is too awkward or if there is doubt as to the professional breach ("Is that student's style of dress too provocative or are you just out of date with acceptable fashion?").

Learners naturally feel aligned with the physician, and some may feel that they can treat the office staff or other hospital professionals as inferior. If this occurs, it needs to be explicitly confronted. Respect for the experience and for the value of the other team members is fundamental for a well-functioning healthcare team. Even if we are short at times of stress with our staff, we have a long-standing relationship into which such (hopefully) occasional excursions take place. We can point out strengths, challenges and boundaries of the relationships we have with our hospital and office staff and role-model them respectfully. Equally, any disrespect we may express to a learner about a colleague is highly infectious and inappropriate. Learners are not our private venting occasions for comments we would not otherwise share. It does not have to be honey, but it should not be vinegar.

Social Challenges

Learners, like physicians, will face social issues in a small community. Discussing these with a learner is important. Meeting patients in public settings, learning not to discuss confidential topics (i.e. all patient–doctor issues) outside of the office, not entering into prohibited personal relationships with patients are all specific learner and teacher issues while they are in your practice. The clinical teacher is often more clued into these issues due to the weight of responsibility they carry with regard to clinical care and social responsibility. These boundaries may not seem as clear to the learner who may relish in the attention they accrue socially in a small community by being associated with the medical staff.

While most learners will find their own happy medium in this regard, others may need direction. Clinical teachers may know some of these lessons implicitly, but may need to make social boundaries explicit for the learner. This takes on more importance in smaller communities where anonymity is non-existent for the medical staff. This is one of the challenges that clinicians experience when practicing in such an environment. It is a good topic for general orientation to what professional life is like in a given community. This might also encompass some of the religious, cultural, social and economic aspects of life in a small town that might not be obvious to the newly arrived learner.

Safety Issues

It can help to tell all learners early on to "listen to their gut," to recognize that "Oh-oh" feeling. Let them know that if they feel uncomfortable with a patient or health professional interaction, they should listen to that. If they feel uncomfortable, they need to ask for assistance, something is not right: they are here to learn, and bumping up against a boundary or limitation is time to call in their supervisor. Part of our role is to teach learners to avoid unsafe situations.

Medical misunderstandings with patients can create problems that will linger or fester, long after the learner has moved on to another rotation. The learner may feel silly saying that they are not comfortable in a given clinical scenario, but this is a powerful teaching and learning moment. It may be an opportunity to deal with learning issues of confidence, attitude or skill level that can often be worked out with a bit of support. The learner needs to work within a certain comfort level to learn and the patient deserves an equally comfortable treatment environment. Dealing with an angry patient, for example, may not be a skill the learner has acquired and it is an intimidating scenario for all of us. Any situation which may escalate to violence must be considered high-risk and carefully dealt with. Both the patient and learner need to feel safe and it is the clinical teacher's role to leave the door open for supporting learners in these times and shoulder the burden themselves when that would be best for the patient or the learner. As with most things in medicine, prevention is better than treatment.

EDUCATIONAL CONSIDERATIONS

Role-modeling relationships and boundaries is thus a necessity in the community learning context. Teaching learners about boundaries can be as simple as describing situations where we feel uncomfortable as clinicians. It can also be as challenging as confronting a learner about inappropriate comments or behavior.

Clinical teachers may not be used to making their implicit knowledge and assumptions explicit for the learner. The counsel of colleagues to bounce our perspective off can help us, as it is natural to want to avoid such explicit discussions. It comes with the teaching territory though, and as in giving effective feedback on other aspects of medical care, a focus on behavior is a good place to start. Some examples that can be used for explicit discussions with learners are illustrated in Table 23.4.

Table 23.4 Sample Scenarios for Discussion with Learners

How can I help?
Your good friend and patient is dying of cancer at home, and is under your care. It is becoming increasingly difficult to achieve optimal pain control.
How do you cope with your friend's needs while dealing with your own grief?
Can't you do something?
Your dear friend is dying of cancer. Your physician spouse is your friend's doctor. You cannot bear to see your friend in pain, and wonder why your spouse cannot better control it.
Conflicting loyalties
You notice that your physician colleague seems stressed and is making some mistakes in medical practice. You are unsure if your colleague considers you to be his personal physician, but you are not aware of him having another physician, and you have written him the occasional prescription for pain medication for his intermittent chronic back pain.
The slippery slope
You are a physician/teacher and you see your current resident at the movies with a hospital nurse who is also a patient in your practice and has seen the resident as a patient.

SUMMARY

Relationship and boundary issues are a large part of the conscious and unconscious sense of being a community physician. Regard for ethical decision-making principles will help the physician recognize high-risk situations, high-risk patients and their own unique vulnerabilities, and thus avoid dysfunctional boundary violations. Providing medical care for patients who know the physician in roles in addition to the patient role is rewarding yet carries challenges. The physician's spouse and family have their own special relationship and medical care issues. Relationship and boundary issues are no less important for our learners and need to be taught by implicit and explicit methods. Community practice is an ideal environment for learners to reflect on and to gain experience with these issues that they themselves will "live" each day in their future work.

FURTHER READING

Dunn SFM, Freeman R. Risky business: teaching about sexual abuse by physicians. *J Aggress Maltreatment & Trauma*. 1997; 1(2): 281–305.

Rourke J, Smith LFP, Brown JB. Patients, friends, and relationship boundaries. *Can Fam Phys*. 1993; 39: 2557–64.

Rourke L, Rourke JTB. Close friends as patients in rural practice. *Can Fam Phys*. 1998; 44: 1208–10.

Websites

CMA Code of Ethics. Canadian Medical Association; 2004. Available at: www. policybase.cma.ca/PolicyPDF/PD04-06.pdf (accessed August 9, 2011).

CPSNL Medical Act 2005 By-law No. 5 (Code of Ethics). Available at: www.cpsnl.ca/ default.asp?com=Bylaws&m=292&y=&id=5 and 2008 Policy on boundary violatins and on misconduct of a sexual nature. Available at: www.cpsnl.ca/default. asp?com=Policies&m=340&y=&id=9 (accessed August 9, 2011).

CPSO. Maintaining Boundaries with Patients. Members' Dialogue. Sept/Oct 2004. Available at: www.cpso.on.ca/uploadedFils/downloads/cpsodocuments/members/ Maintaining%20Boundaries.pdf (accessed August 9, 2011).

LaPuma J, Priest ER. Is there a doctor in the house? An analysis of the practice of physicians treating their own families. *JAMA*. 1992; 267:1810–12. Available at: www.jama. ama-assn.org/cgi/reprint/267/13/1810 (accessed August 9, 2011).

Reilly DR. Not just a patient: the dangers of dual relationships. *CJRM*. 2003; 8(1): 51–3. Available at: www.cma.ca/index.cfm/ci_id/36734/la_id/1.htm (accessed August 9, 2011).

Rourke L. Reflections on finding and keeping balance as a physician. *MUN Student Wellness Newsletter*. Issue 12: May/June 2009. Available at: www.med.mun.ca/Student Affairs/Our-servicess/Student-Wellness/Wellness-Newsletter.aspx (accessed August 9, 2011).

www.pubmedcentral.nih.gov/picrender.fcgi?artid=2278267&blobtype=pdf (accessed August 9, 2011).

24

Preventing Burnout

Karen Trollope-Kumar

JENNIE'S STORY

Jennie is a rural family physician in her 40s, who has always welcomed students into her practice. Often she had a family practice resident, and sometimes a clinical clerk. Now she is being asked to take first-year students as well, for their initial family medicine experience. But this year, she feels strangely reluctant to take on any more students. She returns the request for student placement, saying that she does not want to take students this year. She gets a concerned phone call the next day.

> "But Doctor, you've always taken students! We count on you to take them regularly. Won't you please reconsider?"

Jennie tells the administrator that she will think it over and get back to her. In the lunchroom, she talks it over with one of her colleagues.

"I'm just sick of teaching," she says. "It takes up too much of my clinical time and I get paid very little for it. Also, do you remember that the last resident I had – he kept questioning me about my management plans, asking me if what I was doing was evidence-based? The one before that wrote in my evaluation that I do not spend enough time teaching. And then there was a student last year who had no idea how to talk to patients, and who got one patient so upset that she got up and left the clinic. I just don't have the patience for any of this any more!"

Jennie's story illustrates some of the elements of burnout, specifically with regard to her role as a teacher. Burnout is a form of mental distress that results in decreased work performance, usually arising from a sense of powerlessness, frustration and inability to achieve work goals. Symptoms of burnout include emotional exhaustion, feelings of cynicism and detachment, and a sense of ineffectiveness and lack of personal accomplishment. The condition has been identified in many groups, particularly among people working in service professions such as medicine, teaching, nursing and ministry.

A physician experiencing burnout often reports dissatisfaction with his or her career choice, and patients also are more likely to report dissatisfaction with the care they receive from such a physician. The physician who feels emotionally exhausted tries to cope by distancing himself or herself emotionally from work. However, the resulting feelings of detachment are often linked with a sense of cynicism and ineffectiveness. Job satisfaction and a sense of personal accomplishment decrease.

Other symptoms and signs that can accompany burnout include over-involvement with patients, irritability, sleep problems, poor judgment and interpersonal conflicts. Some physicians experience frequent illnesses, while others may develop addictive behaviors. Often, physicians who describe their own experience of burnout speak about a sense of loss of meaning in their lives, an apathy toward everything that was once rewarding. Physicians seem to be particularly at risk for burnout because of their intense investment in their profession. For some physicians, the triad of doubt, guilt and an excessive sense of responsibility result in neglect of personal and social aspects of life. A self-destructive pattern of overwork can cause havoc in the physician's professional and personal life.

ASSESSMENT

A tool has been developed to measure burnout, called the Maslach Burnout Inventory (MBI) (www.mindtools.com/stress/Brn/BurnoutSelfTest.htm). This is a 22-item questionnaire that evaluates the level of depersonalization, emotional exhaustion and feelings of low personal accomplishment that characterize a state of burnout. The MBI can be a useful tool for the assessment of a physician who may be experiencing the early stages of burnout. Physicians at any age can experience burnout, though studies show that physicians early in their careers are more prone to burnout than mid-career physicians. Physicians who have many other caregiving responsibilities, such as young children or elderly parents, may have more difficulty maintaining a work–life balance and this may contribute to the development of burnout. Though having a family may be stressful, being single has been found to be an independent risk factor for burnout. The choice of career within the medical profession also plays a part. Oncologists appear to be particularly at risk, perhaps because they are constantly exposed to people who are seriously ill or dying. However, palliative care physicians have not been found to be at greater risk for burnout, though their exposure to dying patients is even more. The team environment in which palliative physicians work is considered to be a protective factor.

Physicians who are also teachers must balance complex roles. Often they are teaching within a clinical environment, and they must ensure high-quality care of patients while, at the same time, attempting to provide excellent educational opportunities for students. While physicians have had many years of training for their clinical roles, they may have had little or no training for their teaching role. If the physician-teacher does not have much understanding of teaching methods and learning styles, the task of teaching in clinical settings will likely be less rewarding.

Teacher burnout may arise from the demands placed on the clinician from the teaching role itself. Enrolment in medical schools across the province has been steadily rising over the past few years, and so the demand for clinical placements has also been rising. Busy family physicians often enjoy having a student in the practice, but there can be drawbacks. With a student in the clinic, patient flow in the office may be less efficient. Finding time to teach the student can be very difficult when the physician is coping with the multiple demands of a busy practice. And some students can be challenging!

Another problem identified by physician-teachers is the relative lack of recognition of the teaching role within the medical community. In the university environment, it is often research or administrative roles that are valued more than teaching roles. The busy clinician who is also interested in academic promotion may choose to focus on more highly valued activities to advance his or her career. The teaching role is seldom well remunerated, and this may be another deterrent for potential physician-teachers.

Two of the early symptoms that are warning signs of impending burnout include exhaustion and a sense of cynicism. Exhaustion can result from an excessive work burden or an inability to set appropriate boundaries between work and personal life. Sometimes, a physician's particular skills, talents and interests are not well-matched to the job. Cynicism often sets in when the work load is overwhelming or when there is a clash between personal values and the values of the institution in which the physician works.

In a recent Canadian study, Leiter reported that "values congruence" was a significant predictor of professional efficacy, particularly for women physicians. When physicians experienced congruence of their personal values with the health system in which they worked, they were much less liable to experience distress, even in demanding situations.

PREVENTION

Are physicians who teach more or less susceptible to burnout? Although there are some conflicting reports, more studies suggest that teaching may have a protective role against burnout. Physicians who teach often feel a greater sense of engagement with their work, and job engagement has consistently been shown to protect against burnout. This engagement results from the joy that comes from sharing one's clinical insights and wisdom, the learning that is stimulated by a process of teaching, and positive effects of the teacher–student relationship. In such an environment, cynicism is less likely to take root.

The complex task of balancing clinical and teaching roles must be carefully addressed by the physician-teacher in order to avoid exhaustion, the other precursor to burnout. The individual physician who is trying to balance multiple roles should carefully examine the tasks of his or her working day. What part of the job is providing the greatest satisfaction? Unsatisfying work takes a greater toll on the individual, and job environments in which the physician feels a lack of control are particularly stressful.

Mentorship of physician-teachers by more experienced colleagues is a powerful way to prevent burnout. Mentors can serve as role models, helping their younger colleagues to shape a career that is both personally and professionally satisfying. At times of crisis, a mentor can provide a lifeline to a colleague in distress.

What makes an effective clinical teacher? Some key qualities are outlined in a recent review article by Ramani in *Medical Teacher*. First of all, clinical teachers must have a passion for teaching and be able to share this with their students. They should demonstrate both clinical competence and exemplary human qualities in the clinic and at the bedside. They should understand, and be able to use, a variety of teaching methods, gauging their learners' level of knowledge and matching teaching strategies accordingly. Clinical teachers also need to be able to provide feedback to students in ways that are both affirming and constructive.

Physicians who want to enhance their teaching skills can access many excellent resources on practical teaching tools that are effective in a busy clinical environment. A useful example of such a tool is called the "one minute preceptor," which is a set of micro-skills specifically tailored for the short time available for teaching in the clinic.

Teaching in outpatient and inpatient settings each has its unique challenges. In the outpatient setting, teaching time is often very short and clinicians may be attending to several patients at the same time. In the hospital environment, patients may be too sick to participate in the teaching encounter, and the rapid turnover of patients prevents students from understanding the natural history of the disease. In both environments, clinical care takes priority over teaching. The most successful physician-teachers are able to seamlessly integrate teaching into clinical settings, rather than trying to set aside specific times for teaching.

RECOVERY

How do we protect ourselves against burnout, and how do we recover from it? A recent study by Jensen looked at resilience among family physicians and highlighted the importance of maintaining interest and engagement in one's work, keeping organized and maintaining some control over one's work environment. The family physician respondents in this study also highlighted caring for one's physical health, taking time away from the practice, and paying attention to personal relationships. Those physicians who were able to attend to all these dimensions of their lives reported high levels of job satisfaction.

A recent review article by Kearney in *JAMA* on self-care of physicians offered many strategies that may help to prevent or treat burnout. In this study, health professionals working in palliative care spoke about the importance of spirituality in preventing burnout. The ability to create meaning out of painful or difficult events is a spiritual task, essential for those working with patients who are dying. Physicians who perceived their role in purely biomedical terms were found to be less engaged with patients and less satisfied with their work. Those physicians who considered their role to encompass both biomedical and psychosocial aspects of care found their work very satisfying.

Some practical measures cited in Kearney's article on self-care include: mindfulness meditation, reflective writing, having a supportive work community, managing workload, practicing self-care activities, continuing educational activities, team approaches to stress reduction and the development of self-awareness skills.

Self-awareness in the workplace involves becoming more conscious, not only of the needs of the patient and the work environment, but also of one's own subjective experience. Being aware of one's subjective experience creates space for feelings of compassion towards oneself as well as the patient. The skills of self-awareness can be developed through practices such as mindfulness meditation, which can be used as a tool to promote resilience. Increasing evidence shows that developing self-awareness has a significant protective effect for people working in high-stress environments. While the physician who uses self-care alone may cope by setting limits to his work, the physician who develops self-awareness may become more deeply engaged in the work without becoming exhausted.

Let's return to the situation of Jennie, the rural physician experiencing teacher burnout. Her feelings of apathy and disengagement with the task, as well as the feelings of frustration with the students, are important clues that suggest early burnout. Once she has realized that these feelings are associated with burnout, she could look for specific ways to prevent the problem from getting more severe. Sometimes, it is necessary to take a break from the type of work that is causing the stress. She may be well advised not to take students for a few months, while she gains some perspective on the problem and formulates a plan for change.

During this period of reflection, she may consider what she can control about the situation. Perhaps she prefers residents to first-year students, or vice versa. She could then request that students at that level of training be posted with her. If it is difficult to find the time to teach during a busy afternoon in the office, she may want to attend a continuing medical education event on innovative ways of teaching "on the fly." Such events can be invigorating and allow physicians the opportunity to share problems and solutions with their peers. If the expectations of some students seem unreasonable, she may want to plan some time at the beginning of the rotation to clarify goals with the student.

Doing some reflective writing about her experiences of teaching may be helpful. In this process, she may be able to clarify for herself both the frustrations and the joys of teaching. Sometimes, the onerous aspects of the task can overshadow the joys of the work. By writing about her experiences, she may be able to remind herself of how satisfied she felt when a student learned something significant, and how delighted she was to hear from a student she had taught years earlier.

Jennie should also review her strategies for self-care. Perhaps her frustration with teaching is part of a larger problem with overwork and self-neglect. She may need to review her priorities, and deliberately plan to take more time to care for her physical and emotional self. If she does not feel happy in the practice of medicine, she will not be able to transmit any enthusiasm for the work to her students. Finally, Jennie could reach out to colleagues for support, asking for suggestions about new ways to enjoy her experience as a clinical teacher. If she feels she is entering a depression and the teaching burnout is a symptom, then she may need to discuss this with her physician.

How does a good clinical teacher become a truly excellent teacher? A teacher may have mastered the technical competencies to teach well in the clinical setting. However, the teacher who aims for excellence must also develop emotional and attitudinal competencies, subtle skills such as self-awareness and self-reflection. These exemplary teachers seek out feedback from their students and peers in order to develop their knowledge and hone their teaching skills. They model excellent communication skills and relationships with patients, and they engage in an on-going personal process of self-reflection. This journey towards greater understanding insulates these teachers from burnout in a truly integrated way.

FURTHER READING

Balch C, Copeland E. Stress and burnout among surgical oncologists: a call for personal wellness and a supportive workplace environment. *Ann Surg Oncol.* 2007; **14**(11): 3029–32.

Jensen P, Trollope-Kumar K, Waters H. *et al.* Building physician resilience. *Can Fam Phys.* 2008; **54**: 722–9.

Kearney M, Weininger R, Vachon M, *et al.* Self-care of physicians caring for patients at the end of life. *JAMA.* 2009; **301**(11): 1155–64.

Lee J, Stewart M, Belle Brown J. Stress, burnout and strategies for reducing them: what's the situation among Canadian family physicians? *Can Fam Phys.* 2008; **54**: 234–5.

Leiter M, Frank E, Matthews TJ. Demands, values, and burnout. *Can Fam Phys.* 2009; **55**: 1224–5.

Maslach C, Leiter M. Early predictors of job burnout and engagement. *J Appl Psychol.* 2008; **93**(3): 498–512.

Maslach C, Leiter M. *The Maslach Burnout Inventory.* 3rd ed. Palo Alto, CA: Consulting Psychologists Press. Available at: www.mindtools.com/stress/Brn/BurnoutSelfTest.htm (accessed August 9, 2011).

Neher J, Gordon K, Meyer B, *et al.* A five-step "microskills" model of clinical teaching. *J Am Board Fam Pract.* 1992; **5**: 419–24.

Ramani S, Leinster S. Teaching in the clinical environment. AMEE guide no 34. *Med Teach.* 2008; **30**: 347–64.

Rutter H, Herzberg J, Paice E. Stress in doctors and dentists who teach. *Med Educ.* 2002, **36**: 543–9.

Websites for Teaching and Learning resources

http://creativecommons.org/
http://chec-cesc.afmc.ca/
www.mededworld.org/
http://services.aamc.org/30/mededportal/servlet/segment/mededportal/information/

Websites for Physician Self-awareness and Self-care

www.practitionerrenewal.ca/
www.mindtools.com/stress/Brn/BurnoutSelfTest.htm
www.aachonline.org/events/event_details.asp?id=133309

25

Keeping up with the Literature

Yogi Sehgal

A large part of teaching involves, not only maintaining what we have already learned, but also increasing our skills and knowledge base to mesh with the constantly changing world of medical science. On a weekly basis, it seems, our knowledge of mechanisms of disease and treatments evolve, and in many cases some of the standard treatments of the past become obsolete. Keeping up with these advances is important if we are to be able to share relevant, up-to-date knowledge and skills with learners. In learning how to maintain our lifelong learning skills, we provide our learners with a model of how they can also do this. As well, we demonstrate that learning in medicine is a career-long endeavor, because we cannot know all of it and it is a constantly evolving knowledge base. Maintenance and advancement of our skills and knowledge is an important part of our practice and teaching. What are the barriers to lifelong learning and what are some approaches to work around them?

Most physicians have the skills to find the answer to a specific question. But awareness and questions about new therapies or tests may not even occur to the community-based physician until they are already in regular use. Many physicians simply are not exposed to even a manageable trickle of important new medical information. How can we improve access to continuing medical education and keep ourselves on the leading edge of medical science?

BARRIERS

Technology

Much of our learning nowadays involves use of computers and the internet. Those who either are uncomfortable with or resist use of such technologies are automatically at a disadvantage in maintaining lifelong learning. Is there a way of more easily integrating technology into medical learning?

Time

The reality is that there are only so many hours in the day, and there are only so many hours one wishes to spend doing work. There are already many demands on our work time, including direct patient care, paper or computer work, phone calls, meetings, committee work and teaching. Commuting to and from work or from one site to another, such as going to an elderly patient's home to do a house-call, or going from a clinic to the hospital to see an inpatient are also time-consuming. Where in this mix; do we fit in our own learning?

Access

In rural communities, accessing learning can be a major undertaking. It may involve the logistical difficulties involved in closing down a practice for a few days to attend a conference or the difficulties associated with having a computer system installed to be able to access learning via the internet. In many isolated communities, transportation issues, including weather, can present an extra challenge in attending courses and conferences in person. In some situations, the workplace is not supportive of taking time off to learn.

Cost

Access is also affected directly by cost. Unbiased courses that are not heavily sponsored by parties with conflicts of interest can be prohibitively expensive. Add to that, the lost income from not working while attending such courses and the continued expenses at the office left behind as well as transportation involved in getting there, and the financial barrier is significant. Are there any ways of reducing the cost or at least obtaining the necessary teaching in a more financially efficient manner?

Resistance to Change

For many people, it is difficult to accept that what we have been doing in some circumstances, while adequate for what we knew 20, 10 or even 2 years ago, is no longer adequate for today's understanding of certain problems. In addition, it is a challenge for some physicians to change, given patients' expectations that have been created by years of following the previous standard. It is difficult to be the first person to prescribe a new intervention, but, at the same time, no one wants to be the last one to prescribe an inadequate or inappropriate older intervention. Also, as human beings, we hesitate to change what we perceive has always been working, whether in medicine or in any other facet of our lives. Are there ways of encouraging these changes in subtle ways?

Legal Climate

Sadly, our system does encourage the practice of "defensive medicine," wherein we practice in such a way as to avoid legal actions. In some cases, this prevents us from following the medical evidence until there is a critical mass of colleagues who have endorsed it as well. As a result, another barrier to lifelong learning rears its head: why learn a new intervention when one may not use it in practice? Is there a way to mitigate the effect of defensive medicine?

"MY BRAIN IS FULL" SYNDROME

The vastness of both the basic current fund of medical knowledge, as well as recent and constantly evolving advances in that fund of knowledge, can be overwhelming to many physicians. Even specialists in any particular subspecialty may find this difficult, and they have only to concentrate on one particular subject area. After many years of medical school, one can imagine it being easy to believe that very little more learning could possibly be useful. Is there a way of boiling down this information so it can be efficiently analyzed and used by everyday practicing physicians?

Data Interpretation

For many physicians, the data in medical research are presented with such complexity that the idea of interpreting the data and then putting it into practice is daunting. Even many young physicians who have been trained specifically to critically appraise the medical literature commonly struggle with this. The inherent conflict of interest of authors of papers sponsored by the pharmaceutical industry can leave some physicians treading a fine line between being a sceptic and a cynic. In many situations, the clinical trials present more questions than answers. Are there techniques that might help with data interpretation?

The Religion of Guidelines

Many physicians struggle with guidelines, especially when they conflict with each other. Many guideline authors have connections to the pharmaceutical industry, as well as other conflicts of interest, rendering it a challenge to sort out which ones are reasonable. Guidelines should be treated as suggestions rather than a standard of care but, unfortunately, despite the poor quality of guidelines, many physicians think of them as standards. How can we learn to comfortably practice medicine that may be in conflict to some guidelines?

The Patient as an *n* of 1

It is difficult to balance the evidence in medical literature with individual treatment plans. Patients in our practices are not necessarily the same as in trial populations, so we must find a balance between evidence-based medicine (the results of trials) and eminence-based medicine (what the specialists to whom we might refer will do) and reality. In many cases, the learning needed is going to be experiential as well as experimental. How do we develop the experience to integrate the evidence of medical literature with the reality of medical practice?

There is no Evidence

For many clinical questions, there simply has not been a clinical trial that answers the question, either because the trial has never been attempted, or perhaps because it has not been undertaken in the population of interest, or perhaps there has not been a robust enough trial to answer the question. This can create a feeling of cynicism about the paucity of evidence in the medical literature in general. Frustration can set in if several questions in a row come up with no specific answer from the literature. Is there an approach of what to do when there is little evidence?

STRATEGIES

Despite all the barriers presented above, there are many simple solutions to ease us into the flow of traffic of medical information without taking away significantly from other parts of our work or personal lives.

Technology

For some, technology can be a barrier, while for others, it can also be a very useful tool in maintaining and increasing our competence. Although not 100% essential, getting comfortable with computers, personal digital assistants or the internet are becoming increasingly indispensable in staying up-to-date. Without these tools, it does require more time and effort to stay up-to-date, but it is not impossible. Low-tech physicians who are in the habit of regularly reading select journals will also remain up-to-date and need not change that continuing education strategy if it works for them. Most younger or more technologically savvy practitioners will have access to a wider selection of online resources, but will still need strategies to ensure that this access gets used.

Time

Even with the best technology, we simply do not have enough time to keep up with all of the medical literature. There is too much information for the individual to find, analyze, process and put into practice. How then can we possibly keep up? There are many organizations and services that are able to synthesize this information and present it in a concise format that requires a lot less time and effort to review. Learning time can then better be spent deciding which resources to access. One can access such resources for free or a nominal cost, although some very useful ones can be expensive. In general, however, the cost of such resources is minimal compared with the cost of going to a conference or course, and is usually far more convenient.

Even with resources in place to make learning more efficient, one still needs to set aside some formal time for learning, just as one might set aside time for meetings or committee work. This formalized learning time makes keeping up-to-date simpler, gives it importance in our lives and allows learning in a more relaxed form. This is not essential, as there are ways of integrating learning into other parts of our lives, but common sense dictates that giving it a set time makes it not only more likely to happen, but also to be completed in an efficient manner.

Access

Twenty years ago, there was no simple solution for access. However, nowadays, so many people have been faced with this issue that, even in the most isolated communities, there have been developed methods for accessing information. Mostly this involves the use of the internet, but not exclusively. If, however, we are willing to embrace the various technologies available, then a plethora of low-cost or free resources present themselves at the click of a button. If one is connected to the internet, one can find the answers to specific questions by searching the medical literature directly using PubMed or similar search engines. Alternatively, databases such as Up-To-Date or Cochrane can provide a concise summary of their authors' interpretation of the medical literature on a specific topic.

For those who still do not feel they can feasibly use the internet, there are many resources in published paper form such as ACP Journal Club or the *Medical Letter*, or in the format of spoken word compact discs, such as Primary Care Medical Abstracts or *EMRAP*. These do involve some cost but allow those without computers to still keep up with important advances. The danger of using such publications, however, is that the usefulness of the information does depend on a reliable author who is without bias. For the average practitioner, this is usually a reasonable compromise.

Even with these simple solutions, one might still wonder how to incorporate such learning within our schedules. The advantage of CDs or podcasts is that they can be easily incorporated into other parts of our day. That is, they can be listened to while commuting to and from work or between work sites, or during walks or other long trips. There are even resources that can come directly to the physician. These take less than a minute per day to go through and can be read while doing something menial. Info-POEMS, for example, is a resource that, on an almost daily basis, emails out a brief synopsis of a potentially useful paper and even gives a suggestion of what to do with the results.

Cost

Cost weighs in heavily in everyone's lifelong learning decisions. It is one of the reasons that pharmaceutical companies have been able to successfully incorporate themselves in funded CME sessions when, to any outsider, this funding creates an inherent conflict of interest. Most universities and many governments have understood the importance of making available CME to teachers, so there are many programs to fund access to some of the more costly resources. However, this is variable from school to school and government to government. Some low-cost resources include:

➤ *Podcasts*: These are mostly free or available at a nominal cost. They consist of medical information being recorded in an audio or sometimes in video format by a medical organization such as Therapeutics Education Collaborative or *Annals of Internal Medicine*. Most often, the format consists of a radio-program-like session involving a discussion around either a specific medical issue or a recent issue of a journal. Usually available for direct download from the websites of providers or downloadable through online music stores such as iTunes, these cover a wide range of topics. The quality of these depend on the agenda of the publisher of the podcast, but their low cost and generally reliable sources make medical podcasts a very useful option for many.

➤ *Faculty*: Medical schools often provide their faculty with access to online resources to allow easy access to information for teaching and research. This may come in the simple form of free access to journal articles or may be as comprehensive as giving remote access to databases such as Up-to-Date or Essential Evidence Plus, amongst others.

➤ *Online courses*: There are several randomized trials demonstrating the effectiveness of online learning compared with traditional learning. These are available in a multitude of topics and formats, and have met with mixed success. There are even online problem-based learning groups.

RESISTANCE TO CHANGE

Changing one's own practice in a group setting sometimes necessitates a concomitant change in the practice of one's colleagues' as well. Small-group learning sessions where colleagues learn from each other in a non-stressful setting are one of the ways these subtle changes can be made. McMaster University among others produces quality small-group problem-based learning modules that allow discussion around cases and sharing of evidence, as well as experiences, among colleagues.

LEGAL CLIMATE

The legal system does provide a challenge to lifelong learning and particularly to implementation of new evidence in medicine. On the one hand, standards of care do sometimes lag behind the evidence, so does one follow what had been the standard of care, or what should and soon will be the standard of care based on newer evidence? This is actually a very important reason to stay up-to-date. One needs to be able to have a documented discussion with the patient about what is the standard option and what might be a newer option. As a teacher, it behooves us to at least know what our learners may end up with as their standard of care by the time they are in practice.

"MY BRAIN IS FULL"

There is no need to learn everything there is to know in medicine. It would be an unattainable goal. This is why there are experts and resources out there to answer questions that may come up. Having the humility to admit not knowing something and looking it up only makes one smarter in the long run.

DATA INTERPRETATION

There are some basic skills needed to be able to keep up with medical literature, but they are actually quite simple, and the better learning resources include them in their presentations. Data interpretation starts with a basic understanding of how to properly understand a clinical study.

Patient: (Is my PATIENT similar to those in the study?)
Intervention: (What is the specific INTERVENTION in this trial?)
Comparison: (What COMPARISON is used as the standard?)
Outcome: (What difference would it make to the OUTCOME?)

Once the correct question is formulated, the answer can be determined by looking at the data in simple terms. In reading the literature, absolute or relative-risks or benefits are important concepts for therapeutic interventions, while sensitivity or specificity are relevant for diagnostic interventions.

Absolute-risk would indicate the actual measured differences between the outcomes between the intervention group and the comparison group, whereas relative-risk would be a proportionate difference. For example, imagine a trial where patients without treatment (i.e. treated with a placebo) had a 1% mortality, while those patients given drug A showed better outcomes. In this study, if drug A had a 0.5% mortality one could express it as follows:

	Drug A	Placebo	Absolute Difference	Relative Difference
Mortality	0.5%	1%	0.5% (1.0–0.5%)	50% (0.5/1.0%)

In simple terms, half as many people died with drug A than with placebo (relatively a 50% reduction) whereas there was only a 0.5% actual difference in mortality between the two groups (the absolute difference). One could also express this in the form of "number needed to treat" or NNT. This is the number of people needed to take drug A to have one person benefit from the intervention (i.e. in this case for one person to be saved). This can be calculated by dividing 1 by the absolute difference, in this case 1/(0.5%), which yields a NNT of 200. In other words, 200 people would need to be treated with drug A to save one person's life. This does not sound as impressive as saying that the drug has a 50% relative reduction in mortality. Concepts such as "number needed to treat (or harm)" are easily calculated and give a more balanced clinical perspective.

Sensitivity and specificity tend to confuse people. In simple terms, sensitivity is the chance that a test will pick up all of the disease in the population, and specificity is the percentage of healthy people who are correctly identified as not having the disease. So an ideal test would have a high sensitivity (i.e. would not miss people who have the disease) and a high specificity (i.e. would not incorrectly call someone as having the disease when they in fact are normal). Once these basic concepts are understood, most practitioners can quickly scan the medical literature for needed information.

The Religion of Guidelines

Guidelines must be taken with a grain of salt, as they do entirely depend on the bias of the guideline-makers and on the population for which they specifically are designed. However, there are some advantages to looking at what some researchers have concluded from looking at the vastness of the evidence on some topics. National physician colleges often have databases of guidelines on a multitude of relevant subjects.

The Patient as an *n* of 1

In reality, staying up-to-date is only as useful as the ability to discuss the information with the patient in order to make an informed decision about an intervention. Some patients want actual numbers while others just want advice. Bringing up the latest information in front of the patient is one way of potentially increasing the therapeutic relationship with a patient, and a way of teaching learners about integrating evidence into practice.

When to Act When There is No Evidence or No Time to Find It?

There are many settings where there is no evidence in the medical literature to answer the clinical question at hand. However, this does not mean that there is no evidence on which we can base our clinical decision-making and our teaching. Evidence can come in many forms, from a large randomized controlled trial to 20 years of clinical experience to solid theory and common sense. There are also situations when physicians have to act before the evidence is known. In many situations, common sense is good enough. The following four principles can guide us in deciding to use a new intervention without good evidence:

1 the intervention makes theoretical sense
2 it is a relatively harmless intervention
3 there is at least theoretically a potentially large benefit
4 the alternative to doing nothing is very often a very bad outcome.

This is not a replacement for good evidence, but can help keep us out of trouble and from jumping into unnecessary new interventions when the evidence is not yet known.

SUMMARY

Keeping up with relevant medical developments is an on-going lifelong enterprise. Often students will be more up-to-date in some areas than we are. This both levels the playing field and reinforces to the student that none of us know it all. This may help them realize that learning is something the teacher and learner have in common.

FURTHER READING

Abdolrasulnia M, Collins BC, Casebeer L, *et al*. Using email reminders to engage physicians in an internet-based CME intervention. *BMC Med Educ*. 2004; **29**(4): 17.

Chan DH, Leclair K, Kaczorowski J. Problem-based small-group learning via the internet among community family physicians: a randomized controlled trial. *MD Comput*. 1999; **16**(3): 54–8.

Davis L, Copeland K. Effectiveness of computer-based dysphagia training for direct patient care staff. *Dysphagia*. 2005; **20**(2): 141–8.

Macrae EM, Regehr G, McKenzie M, *et al*. Teaching practicing surgeons critical appraisal skills with an internet-based journal club: a randomized, controlled trial. *Surg*. 2004; **136**(3): 641–6.

Sargeant J, Curran V, Jarvis-Selinger S, *et al*. Interactive on-line continuing medical education: physicians' perceptions and experiences. *J Contin Educ Health Prof*. 2004; **24**(4): 227–36.

Stewart M, Marshall JN, Østbye T, *et al*. Effectiveness of case-based on-line learning of evidence-based practice guidelines. *Fam Med*. 2005; **37**(2): 131–8.

Taylor RS, Reeves BC, Ewings PE, *et al*. Critical appraisal skills training for healthcare professionals: a randomized controlled trial, *BMC Med Educ*. 2004; **4**(1): 30.

Websites

therapeuticseducation.org
essentialevidenceplus.com
www.ccme.org
www.uptodate.com

26

Generalism and Community-based Medical Education

Keith MacLellan

A QUICK QUIZ

Name an occupation that:
➤ is the one of oldest in the world (not that one, please!)
➤ is absolutely key to the propagation, survival and health of the human race
➤ whose practitioners rely on general, even amateurish training, working in loose partnerships and groups the rules of which have been set since the beginning of time and passed down through generations
➤ the practitioners of which have, as resources, both specialists and spiritual advisers to help, but not dictate, questions of life, death, healthy development, mental and physical well-being and all the crucial factors in a human life.

The answer, of course, is parenthood. But how is it that all societies trust what is arguably the most important job in life to mere jacks-of-all-trades, or generalists, who have no formal, standardized, nationally and internationally accredited specialized training? Animals do the same, presumably relying on instincts. Humans also learn child rearing by direct observation, historical patterns and instinct. But surely human civilization has progressed enough not to rely on intellectually vague concepts such as instinct when raising children? Is it not the human intellect that separates us from animals and has the human intellect not enabled the wonders of technology and progress in general? Why then have we not learned to become specialized and then subspecialized in all aspects of that most important of human activities, parenting? Granted, we can call on a host of sometimes dubious specialists to advise a parent on certain decisions to be made in certain areas and at certain times of a child's life. Similarly, and often as dubious, there are innumerable spiritual and artistic experts whose advice a parent can seek. But where are the truly specialized and thorough parenting courses? Most parents have little idea what they are getting into when deciding to raise a child, despite the work being so crucial on the personal and species levels.

So, why do we choose "generalists" for parenting when, in this day and age, it would certainly be possible to specialize this occupation? This chapter will examine the nature of a generalist's work. We will concentrate in the medical field, and especially in rural medicine where generalism has been the absolute *"sine qua non"* method of practice in any rural area of any country in any century – and will continue to be no matter what technology may have to offer in the future. Medical generalism should not be like parenthood, of course – the example was meant to underline how we do not trust all we do to specialists, even if given the choice. We will see later how medical generalism, unlike parenting, must include mandatory proof of competencies in skillsets shared with specialists.

Another example might be more pertinent to medical generalism. Think of it – within a decade or so there could be a manned expedition to Mars. The crew and the ship will be marvels of technology and specialization, the best human minds can put together. But the trip will take about 21 months and one of the crew will necessarily be a physician. But what kind of physician should be on the mission to Mars? Even backed by robot technology, the best of specialists on Earth and wonderful communication technology, the only choice still will certainly be a superbly trained generalist. In fact, there are many broadly skilled physicians working in rural parts of the world who could qualify right now. Without a doubt, the Mars expedition physician must be trained much of the time in rural areas by community-based training.

It is fair to say medical generalism is threatened and diminishing, at least in so-called "developed" countries. This has been recognized by many national medical organizations, some of which have issued calls in one form or the other to "promote generalism," despite the contrary trend to identify family medicine itself as a specialty.

Perhaps a deeper look at what the term "generalist" really means could help make the rather vague calls to promote generalism a little more practical. Community-based medical education can be a powerful agent for clearing some of the haze around what is meant by the term "medical generalist." Properly done research, founded in community-based teaching and examining typical rural healthcare models, could bring lessons of great benefit to an entire health system under stress, where the escalating inexorable sub-differentiation of work is a major driver of costs and fragmentation, at least in affluent countries.

We will examine two inter-related topics:

1   What is work place "generalism?" Why is it needed in rural areas? What important principles underlie generalism, as applied specifically to medicine? How can it be supported and taught?

2   How, historically and politically, does community-based teaching fit into our traditional medical teaching system? What are the characteristics of the current system for training of physicians? How can community-based medical education promote the generalism so essential for serving any significant and scattered rural/remote populations?

PRINCIPLES OF GENERALISM

As societies become more densely populated, the work of their members becomes more differentiated. Similarly, the more affluent a society, the more it can afford to apportion the labor into smaller and more specialized tasks, those tasks being carried out, of course, by narrowly trained specialists – the more specialized the better.

And why should it not be so? The intellect solves a multitude of problems. Human kind has made enormous advances simply because we have learned to use our minds to break large problems into smaller ones, thereby allowing us to apply smaller specialized bits of knowledge, then joining the bits together to present elegant and useful solutions to a question or task. It is impossible to imagine how else, say, an airplane could be built, or the computer, or any other example of human progress including the conduct of the battle against disease.

The human intellect is a great differentiator. This ability to compartmentalize and specialize is a powerful tool. On the other hand, another quality lies within the human mind. Call it what you will – Soul, Spirit, God, Art – but this force is a great integrator. This is what gives humans the ability to bring things together, to make sense under a higher order, to allow flow, resolution, even redemption. Taking things apart and bringing things together. Nature has both.

There are many ways to look at this but, to take a linear analysis, all humans have the integrating Spirit at one pole and the differentiating, specialized Intellect at the other, both in constant tension (*see* Figure 26.1). Over centuries,

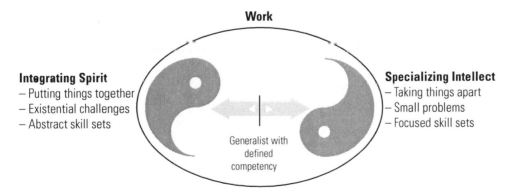

Figure 26.1 Spirit – Intellect Continuum

these poles have become increasingly separated and the tension between them arguably tighter. There are also many ways of looking at this tension in understanding the human condition. What characterizes a true generalist within this framework? The meaning of generalism becomes clearer when we introduce this human spectrum with its opposing poles into any work situation. This brings us to the first principle of generalism.

1 The generalist is NOT the opposite of the specialist
Rather, the generalist is somewhere on the tension spectrum between the intellect and the spirit, between the integrator and the differentiator. Where exactly on that spectrum the generalist can be found varies minute by minute, day by day and week by week, depending on a host of factors. One can imagine the generalist at one time much closer to passion and, at others, almost coldly logical.

So far, this situation would describe just about any human being. But now place this whole spectrum with its opposite poles, and an individual in varying locations along the spectrum, and introduce it into a work situation. It can be almost any kind of work – digging a trench, designing a car, making a sculpture, composing a song, caring for sick humanity. Depending on the task, one would ideally want the worker to be closer to one pole or the other. So, independent of the type of work, how would one identify the true generalist from any working human being? This brings us to our second principle:

2 The generalist must have defined competencies
"Competencies" means what it says – the tasks carried out must be at the same standards as those carried out by a specialist. That is, the competency must have similar outcomes and complications whether performed by a generalist or by a specialist. This also mandates the tasks done by the generalist being recognized as valid and competent by some national standard setting body and, implicitly, by the specialists who "own" that specialized piece of knowledge/capabilities.

"Defined" means two things: 1. defined by the needs of the community; and 2. defined by the common practice of generalist rural peers. Naturally, the competencies would not be the entire set of knowledge/capabilities of a specialist in that field but, instead, a varying sub-set of skills delineated, capably transmitted, permitted and shared. This is nothing new – over the centuries most rural care has been able to function only because, in the absence of specialists, some generalists have learned to perform extremely competently certain procedures or have certain clinical knowledge usually in the domain of specialists. One great threat to rural healthcare is that this has never been formalized and recognized.

The concept of community plays a far greater role for its rural members than for their urban counterparts. Rural communities are diverse for many reasons, including geography, demography, proximity to urban centers, local infrastructure, transport facilities and so on. The needs of a rural community also vary immensely from one to the other. Another characteristic of rural communities is that there are far more people with several different jobs than there are in urban areas. There is, therefore, a greater need for generalists in all forms of labor in rural communities. The rural community workforce is much more vulnerable to the loss of one worker, since the loss of one generalist with several defined competencies, whether by death, relocation or the advent of a specialist, may result in the community losing several capabilities.

For example, a car mechanic in a small town may also be the local locksmith and, say, operate a backhoe. If a franchise oil-changing business sets up shop, the mechanic will lose a major source of income and may be forced to move. The town will then have specialized oil changing, but no longer have backhoe or locksmith services.

In rural healthcare, there are no dedicated autism psychologists, for example. Neither do we find dedicated sports physiotherapists nor social workers who care only for abused women. Nurses work in the Emergency Room one day and in the obstetrics case room the next. Loss of any one nurse, physiotherapist, social worker or psychologist can bring to a halt a host of disparate services. The situation with rural physicians is similar, but perhaps more acute given the nature of the work. Most rural physicians who work in a hospital form spontaneously into teams. The nature of these rural physician teams has not changed much over the centuries. The best functioning teams have a basic skill level in a number of fields that everyone shares (office, ER, OBS, inpatients). There will then be any number of physicians who have acquired extra, more specialized, competencies, usually graded to fit the needs of a community. Surgery, anesthesia and cesarean section capabilities are the three pillars that hold up the rural hospital. The loss of any one pillar, sooner or later, will lead to collapse of the hospital into primary care, triage, geriatrics and palliative care. But rural physicians routinely assume many more defined competencies, such as fracture management, colposcopy, ultrasound, echocardiography, hand surgery, etc. Members of the rural healthcare team are constantly varying from the primary, secondary, and sometimes tertiary, level of care, often hour by hour during their working day. Another threat to rural healthcare is that the grading of competencies to the needs of a community has never been formalized.

Meanwhile, the urban, and especially the academic, medical system is inexorably sub-differentiating. Urban family practice is rarely situated in hospitals or the ER, nor does one find family practitioners doing extra skills of surgery or anesthesia. Primary care is being encroached upon by protocol-driven nurse practitioners, specialized nurses and physician assistants. Losing ground in broad primary care, the urban family practice movement is now itself subspecializing, with a growing number of "special interest" family physicians seeking recognition for full-time non-generalist work. The situation in the certified specialist field is farther along, as general surgeons, internists, psychiatrists give way to sub-subspecialists in the chosen fields. This trend is one of the greatest cost drivers of a medical system. Furthermore, the age-old proven relationship between the generalist and the specialist is now reversing. This brings us to the third principle of generalism:

3 The specialist (and the spiritual/artistic practitioner) exist to serve the generalist

Sir William Osler synthesized thousands of years of medicine. His principles still hold sway in this age of technology. In essence, Osler stated that the only practitioner who was suited to serve sick, suffering humanity was the generalist. His many quotes pleaded with medical students to at least begin practice as generalists and, if possible, to continue as generalists. The so-called "coal face" of medicine, with its undifferentiated presentation of disease, its uncertainties, with the full wind of patient anxiety, trouble and grief blowing strongly against the practitioner, only makes the fog at the face of disease thicker. The needs of patients for guidance, reassurance and clinical acumen, particularly at the rawest and earliest presentation, require a generalist to be present and first in charge. This generalist could call on his own resources or those of his colleagues at either end of the intellect/spirit spectrum: from the purest intellectual or reasoned end of the spectrum for short, sharp, clear specialized intervention and advice; or the generalist could call for advice from the other end of the spectrum – spiritual, artistic or emotional intervention. But it should always be such that practitioners at the poles of the spectrum are there at the call of the generalist, not the other way around.

Since, by definition, generalists do not know everything about every subject, they are true jacks-of-all-trades. The corollary is that they are masters of none. "Knowledge a mile wide but an inch deep" as it is sometimes put. So, in this age of explosion of medical knowledge, does Osler's dictum still hold true or is generalist care now second best? Is generalism simply a sometimes needed but, at its roots, a negative aberrancy, only good enough to be practiced where there are no specialists? Shouldn't more and more patients in need of secondary level care simply be transported? Can telemedicine bridge the gap? Why not replace all generalists with cheaper and more effective non-physicians who can manage chronic disease and triage to the specialist at the secondary care level?

There are insufficient answers in the research literature to address these questions. One could as easily ask whether care closer to home is clinically better and still find few answers. There is evidence that highly skilled procedures, such as coronary artery by-pass grafting, certain vascular surgery, endoscopic retrograde cannulation of the bile duct, do better with higher volume of procedures. It becomes much harder to demonstrate such an effect for many more common procedures and, as in the case of obstetrics, better outcomes are seen with properly screened local care. Transport is not always possible for weather or personnel issues. Where it is possible, one must remember that sending patients elsewhere frequently degrades the local hospital's capabilities to handle, not just the condition for which the patient is being transported, but a host of related conditions as well. The same holds true for telemedicine, where paradoxical degradation of the local hospital's capabilities can frequently be the end result. The problem is that there really has not been much rural-relevant research done to answer these and other questions. Is being born and later dying within an individual's own community important for the definition and support of a rural community? The answer must obviously be "yes". But can this be done properly with generalist care, given the way obstetrics and palliative care are now specializing? With all these silos and sub-silos in the medical system, and with the dearth of rural-relevant research, how is one to assure and support defined competencies, and thus generalism, in rural healthcare?

One relatively new initiative and a hopeful one at that, is community-based medical education. But before we look at this, we must understand how the medical education system functions, what influences and restrictions does it bear, and how it can change.

ACADEMIA, GENERALISM AND COMMUNITY-BASED TEACHING

One fundamental principle underlies all universities since their medieval beginnings in Bologna, Paris and Oxford: "academic freedom;" meaning freedom from political influence, freedom to pursue knowledge wherever it can be found and independent of societal influences, including usefulness to society. One can easily see why academic freedom is so important to universities and their pursuit of knowledge. It is simply unacceptable that some royal entity in the past, or an elected minister of education or health in the present, or some religious leader at any time in present or past, dictate who will be allowed to work in universities and what type of research should be done. However, for many reasons, not the least being that most universities depend primarily on public money to function, the last few decades have seen the rise of a global movement to promote "social responsibility" within universities. Internationally, this has given rise in Europe to the "Bologna Declaration" and more widespread in the world, the "Magna Charta Universitatum" which, while setting academic freedom and prohibiting political interference in its first principles, goes on to declare: ."..peoples and states should become more aware than ever of the part that universities will be called upon to play in a changing and increasingly international society ...". Now signed by over 600 universities, this movement has quite naturally attracted the attention of Canadian universities who have begun their own processes to become more "socially responsible."

University accreditation processes vary country by country but, in medical education, accreditation has been heavily influenced by the Flexner Report of the early 20th century in the USA. At that time, there was a plethora of self-proclaimed "medical schools" turning out physicians and surgeons with skimpy standards for the teaching of their students. Flexner essentially justified, and later enforced, the closure of any medical school in North America that could not show a clear vector between the research lab and the patient's bedside. He was opposed by many of the great clinicians of the day, such as Osler and Peabody, who worried about the demise of purely clinical medicine under the Flexner requirements but who nevertheless lived to witness the growth of prestigious academic health sciences centers in their own clinical backyards. Embers of this situation persist to this day in many Faculties of Medicine, where one of the favored past times of the academic staff is to seek "protected time." Protected from what? Why, from teaching and clinical duties of course. Community-based medical teachers should take note.

The job of accrediting how well Faculties of Medicine are doing in maintaining teaching standards varies country to country, but generally lies in national accrediting colleges, the members of which are, of course, by and large academics. A few countries, primarily for historical reasons, labor under the unfortunate situation of having Faculties of Medicine responsible not just for undergraduate training of medical students but also for postgraduate training of specialists and family physicians. This has the advantage of medical student and Family Medicine resident teaching being vetted by a team that can include a proportion of practicing non-academic family physicians. In practice, the disadvantages of attempting to accredit postgraduate medical programs according to academic, research-based standards in what is essentially a non-research "trade" such as family medicine or surgery can cause severe strain in the system – more so if it involves concepts somewhat new to universities, such as "community" or "population needs".

Whatever the accreditation process, there are many other confounding challenges that universities, and faculties of medicine in particular, face in dealing with a large set of community-based teachers. Governments, for example, might question why they must fund universities to teach, when they then must fund a completely different community-based system to actually do much of the teaching. In some cases, government-funded community teaching actually began from community pressure for recruitment and retention of physicians, then evolved into facilitating the teaching of medical students and residents as one tool for recruitment. Thus, community-based teaching programs often precede any formal university involvement in the community. In the past, faculties of medicine passively passed students and residents "into the boonies" with little understanding of, hope for, or interest in what learning outcomes might ensue.

When government funding and more goal-directed directives begin to flow, universities might make a case for being "community capable" and to seek some of that funding. Part of the problem for governments interested in helping rural communities is that there are few, often no, accountable rural agencies that can accountably accept large funding and initiatives. It has been much easier for governments to give the funding to universities and let it "trickle down." John Kenneth Galbraith, the noted economist, is well known for pointing out that "trickle down" economics made as much sense as a farmer sowing his fields by feeding oats to his horses and turning them loose. We have already seen the importance community plays in rural areas and how diverse one from the other each rural community is in its health and labor needs. This includes the importance of "generalism" in the rural labor market, including the health field.

Can universities sow these rural fields appropriately according to individual community needs? Are universities capable of developing a robust, responsive community capacity or would this actually constitute a threat to the academic freedom so fundamental to all the faculties within a university? Can these community teachers, in the main non-research based, be accepted and welcomed into the traditional ranks of academia?

The answer must be: perhaps. But to do so, Faculties of Medicine must assume some tortuous positions. One way for service to the rural community to solidify within faculties of medicine would be if the faculties were able to show to accrediting bodies that they are building visible means of promoting sustainable generalism, so essential for rural health, to flourish within their naturally hyper-differentiating, intellectual, research-directed internal imperatives. Faculties of Medicine would need to become the principal agents for bringing out from under the table and legitimizing what has gone on for centuries in rural areas – the competent performance of specialized skill sets by generalist physicians. For example, if the concept of "defined competencies" as proposed above is accepted as key to the implementation of generalism, then each department of any faculty of medicine wishing to be community responsive would have to build a demonstrable ability to deliver defined competencies to practitioners whose community has been shown by some acceptable process to require the skill set. A surgeon in training would be able to learn a defined skill set in orthopedics; a family physician would be able to do formal echocardiograms, and so on. This would mean that the national accrediting framework must require a formalized process for promoting defined competencies. The faculties of medicine and accrediting bodies would also have to become involved in the elaboration of national standards of community needs evaluation, competency, regulation and clinical guidelines – big risks, to be sure, and certainly foreign to many academic faculties.

Should the accrediting system be unwilling or unable to formalize and actually effectively promote generalism and defined competencies within each department of each faculty of medicine, there is always the possibility of establishing a national autonomous accrediting body for rural health. This approach, like many others, is essentially a political decision and may be lobbied for by rural communities who feel underserved.

Another possible solution would be to build a medical school from scratch, one that deliberately has built-in community capacity and responsibility. This could be done on a regional scale with at least a measure of selective "adjustment" of accrediting criteria. Such an approach, done properly, could make a definite improvement in clinical care in many communities, particularly if it was mandated to rely on non-academic community physicians "gearing up" their knowledge to teach much of even the basic sciences to medical students. One could predict that generalism and defined competencies would be much easier to incorporate into the formal processes of such a medical school.

Perhaps the most likely scenario is that, after the publication of multiple reports from multiple funded committees, the faculties of medicine will not find it possible to change much at all. Then community-based teaching may be the only hope that generalism will continue to exist to serve rural populations. As it develops, more and more teaching will be done in communities, to the point where at some time or another there will be more local community capacity building. The recruitment by universities of former community-based generalists to administer its programs is occurring in many places, so slow improvement of the lot of the generalist within universities is perhaps inevitable, at least to a point.

ADVICE FOR THOSE INTERESTED IN PROMOTING GENERALISM POLITICALLY

➤ As much as possible, build community capacity. This means establishing definitions of what your local community needs and then setting up some accountable system to receive funding.
➤ Support existing and long-standing community-based teaching programs – try not to let their funding go to faculties of medicine, despite what may be said about accreditation standards.
➤ Bring together existing and long-standing community-based teaching programs in a national manner for their own self-support and exchange of ideas.
➤ Support any regional rural community-based faculty of medicine.
➤ Encourage all faculties of medicine to make appointments of community generalists within and outside of their own structure.
➤ Support any measure which makes community-based teaching easier and simpler.

➤ Keep rural hospitals going with the production and support of at least GP anesthesiologists, GP surgeons and cesarean section capability.
➤ Support any national organization of generalist community rural physicians.
➤ Make "defined competencies" a phrase of common parlance and a concept to be embraced by any teaching or accrediting body.

HELPFUL POINTS FOR THE INDIVIDUAL RURAL GENERALISTS

➤ Seek the support and inspiration of fellow generalists.
➤ Listen to your community's needs and seek out defined competencies wherever they can be found.
➤ Go to specialists and ask them what they find boring and repetitious in their work. Then, if it is a community need, ask to be taught that.
➤ Promote local medical research.
➤ Form as productive and helpful relationships as possible with your faculties of medicine; understand their limitations and take the long view.
➤ Teach the value and fun of a generalist practice with its defined competencies to as many students and residents as possible.

Community-based medical education is a point of focus for political, academic and philosophical perspectives and responses to societal needs. We have an opportunity to get it right and learn from both our past experience and from the communities we are meant to serve.

Index